Weight Management and Obesity

Weight Management and Obesity

Courtney Winston Paolicelli

MOMENTUM PRESS HEALTH

MOMENTUM PRESS, LLC, NEW YORK

Weight Management and Obesity

First published in 2016 by
Momentum Press, LLC
222 East 46th Street, New York, NY 10017
www.momentumpress.net

ISBN-13: 978-1-60650-763-6 (paperback)
ISBN-13: 978-1-60650-764-3 (e-book)

Momentum Press Nutrition and Dietetics Practice Collection

Cover and interior design by Exeter Premedia Services Private Ltd., Chennai, India

First edition: 2016

10 9 8 7 6 5 4 3 2 1

Printed in the United States of America.

I would like to dedicate this textbook to two incredible men: Brent'on S. Winston and Mark A. Paolicelli. Brent'on, even at a young age, you were my inspiration. I hope you find this textbook safe, effective, and fun. Mark, thank you for always being supportive of my nutrition endeavors and my culinary experiments; however, I'm not giving up on the kale chips. Bub and Moose, I love you both.

Abstract

Five decades ago, the major nutrition-related issues facing the United States were nutrient deficiencies, underconsumption of calories, and malnutrition. In 2016, however, the food landscape is drastically different, and today, the United States faces nutrition-related issues more closely associated with over consumption of calories, bigger waistlines, and chronic disease. Overweight and obesity now afflict the majority of U.S. adults and a large percentage of U.S. children. In addition, diet-related chronic diseases that used to be exclusively observed among adults (e.g., cardiovascular disease, type 2 diabetes mellitus, and hypertension) are now being detected in children and adolescents.

To lower the risk and/or assist with the management of chronic illnesses, overweight and obese patients are frequently advised to lose weight. Although there are many proposed "quick fixes" for weight loss, long-term weight management is a struggle for most patients. As such, nutrition and healthcare clinicians need to understand the etiology of weight gain and the science-based steps necessary for proper and adequate weight management interventions.

This textbook comprehensively examines the treatment of overweight and obesity using an individualized approach. Interventions including diet and behavioral modification, pharmacotherapy, surgery, and physical activity are discussed in the context of an overall lifestyle approach to weight management. Characteristics of successful weight management programs are explored, and example menu plans are provided.

Keywords

binge eating disorder, body mass index, calorie balance, cognitive restructuring, dietary guidelines for Americans, empty calorie foods, laparoscopic adjustable gastric banding, laproscopic sleeve gastrectomy, low-carbohydrate diet, low-fat diet, motivational interviewing, obesity, overweight, roux-en-Y gastric bypass, very low-calorie diet

Contents

Acknowledgments xi

Chapter 1 Fundamentals of Nutrition, Calorie Balance, and Body Weight 1
Chapter 2 Epidemiology and Health Consequences of Obesity 11
Chapter 3 Factors Contributing to Overweight and Obesity 23
Chapter 4 Nutrition Assessment 41
Chapter 5 Weight Loss Intervention: Program Characteristics and Components 69
Chapter 6 Weight Loss Intervention: Goal Setting 79
Chapter 7 Weight Loss Intervention: Energy and Macronutrient Approaches to Calorie Reduction 91
Chapter 8 Weight Loss Intervention: Basic Concepts for Nutrition Education 111
Chapter 9 Weight Loss Intervention: Behavior Modification 127
Chapter 10 Weight Loss Intervention: Medications 145
Chapter 11 Weight Loss Intervention: Weight Loss Surgery 157
Chapter 12 Physical Activity 177

Index 185

Acknowledgments

I would like to acknowledge the guidance and assistance provided by my dear friend and colleague, Katie Clark Ferraro. Katie, without your assistance, I would have never gotten through the process of writing this textbook. I truly appreciate your direction, patience, and support.

CHAPTER 1

Fundamentals of Nutrition, Calorie Balance, and Body Weight

Weight management and obesity prevention are two of the hottest topics in health and nutrition today. Clinicians from virtually every medical field seek information on these topics, in part, because of the vast number of patients who have an abnormal or undesirable weight status. This chapter will provide an overview of calorie balance and the macronutrients that contribute to energy intake.

Calorie Balance

Body weight is primarily determined by a simple concept known as energy balance. Energy balance is the ratio of energy ingested through foods and beverages to the energy expended through basal metabolism, the thermic effect of food, and physical activity.

The energy discussed in nutrition and weight management is measured in kilocalories (kcal). One kcal is defined as the amount of heat, or energy, necessary to raise 1 kg of water by 1°C. Although the scientifically correct term for this energy is kcal, most consumer-facing and educational resources refer to this energy as simply calories. For this reason, nutrition facts labels will display energy in terms of calories per serving and calories from fat, as opposed to using kcal.

Energy Ingested

Energy, or calories, ingested by human beings comes from four macronutrients: carbohydrate, fat, protein, and alcohol. Based on its corresponding chemical structure, each of these macronutrients will provide a particular level of energy, or calories, per gram ingested.

Carbohydrates and protein are the least energy-dense of the macronutrients, providing ~4 kcal/g. Alcohol provides 7 kcal/g. Fat is the most energy-dense providing ~9 kcal/g.

The caloric content of foods and beverages is based on the grams of carbohydrate, fat, protein, and alcohol in the associated product. For example, if a food's nutrition facts label states that it has 25 g of carbohydrate (CHO), 1 g of fat (FAT), 1 g of protein (PRO), and no alcohol per single serving, then one serving of that food should have ~113 kcal (although, due to the rounding of some of these numbers, the label may state that the caloric content is slightly higher or lower than this number). See Figure 1.1 for another example of these calculations.

Please note that the U.S. Food and Drug Administration, the agency that oversees nutrition facts labels, allows food manufacturers to round their numbers on the nutrition facts labels. As such, the calculations

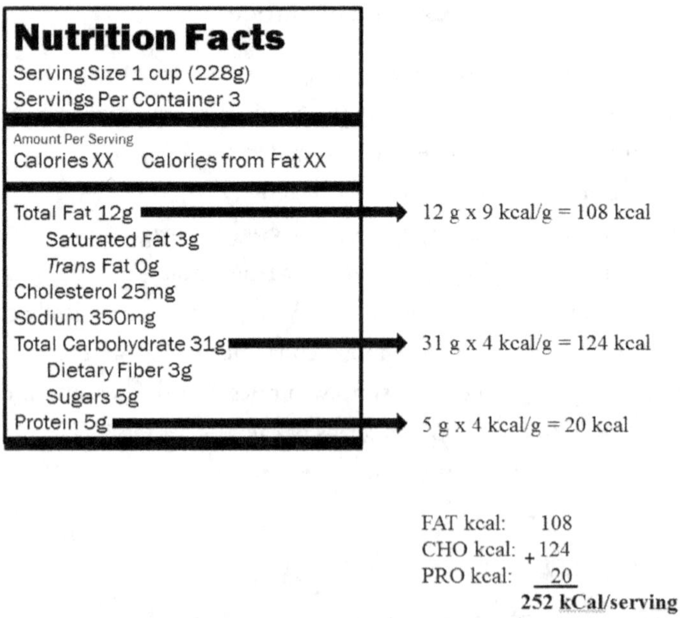

Figure 1.1 The Nutrition Facts Label can be used to estimate the number of calories in one serving of a food item

performed in the examples above may be slightly different from the numbers appearing on the label itself. In addition, the labeling rules for alcohol-containing products are different from nonalcoholic products; therefore, traditional nutrition facts labels may not be available on all alcohol-containing products.

Carbohydrates

Carbohydrates and carbohydrate-containing foods are extremely important to the American diet. In general, most Americans consume plenty of carbohydrates each day; however, the types of carbohydrate-containing foods Americans typically eat are not considered to be ideal. As such, when discussing weight management and obesity prevention, it is imperative to discuss carbohydrates and carbohydrate-containing foods in order to better understand what dietary modifications should be made.

Chemically speaking, carbohydrates are made up of single or strands of carbon rings, called saccharide polymers. These polymers take on four different forms: a single saccharide polymer (monosaccharides), two polymers attached to each other (disaccharides), three to nine polymers in a single strand (oligosaccharides), or ten or more polymers in a single strand (polysaccharides).

Monosaccharide and disaccharide polymers are commonly referred to as simple carbohydrates or simple sugars. Monosaccharide polymers include the most elemental forms of carbohydrate found in nature: glucose, galactose, and fructose. Disaccharide polymers are made up of two monosaccharide polymers joined together, and the three disaccharides are sucrose (glucose + fructose), lactose (glucose + galactose), and maltose (glucose + glucose).

On the nutrition facts label, the monosaccharide and disaccharide content of a food will be indicated on the rows labeled "Total Sugars." It is important to note that total sugars include both the naturally occurring simple sugars (e.g., lactose in milk) and added sugars that are incorporated during food processing (e.g., high fructose corn syrup in ketchup). Future labeling regulations may require manufacturers to distinguish between natural and added sugars, but as of the writing of this book, the current nutrition facts label combines these two sugars.

Oligosaccharide and polysaccharide polymers contain three or more monosaccharide units; thus they are referred to as the complex carbohydrates. Oligosaccharides, which contain three to nine monosaccharide polymers, are commonly found in legumes. Polysaccharides, the longest chains of saccharide polymers, are often called starch and are commonly found in starchy vegetables (e.g., potatoes and peas) and grains (e.g., breads, pasta, and rice).

According to the Institute of Medicine's Dietary Reference Intakes, carbohydrates should make up about 45 to 65 percent of the calories in the diet. Healthy adults should consume a minimum of 130 g of carbohydrates per day, although there are some lower-carbohydrate diets that discourage carbohydrate consumption at this level.

Fats

Dietary fats are an essential component of any health diet. Although dietary fat gained a negative connotation in the 1990s and early 2000s, researchers have shown fat to be a key element in weight management. Fat is known as one of the dietary components that leads to satiety, or feelings of fullness after a meal. Fat also contributes to food's palatability and desirable texture. Nonetheless, when talking about fat, clinicians should realize that not all fats are created equal. Some fats appear to have more health consequences than others. As such, patients should be careful and primarily focus on consuming the healthier fats.

Dietary fats basically fall into three main categories: unsaturated, saturated, and *trans*. Unsaturated fats are made up of carbon chains containing at least one double bond. Monounsaturated fats contain just one double bond, while polyunsaturated fats contain multiple double bonds. Saturated fats do not contain any double bonds and are simply long chains of carbon linked solely by single bonds. *Trans* fats are similar to unsaturated fats in that they do contain at least one double bond; however, they also undergo a configuration change in processing that causes their corresponding *cis* configuration to be altered to a *trans* configuration.

It is important to recognize that foods are typically made up of a combination of fats and rarely contain one single type of fat. For example, olive oil is commonly referred to as a good source of monounsaturated fat; however, it also contains a small amount of saturated fat. Similarly, lard is commonly referred to as a source of saturated fat, but it also contains some monounsaturated fats and polyunsaturated fats.

Not all dietary fats are created equal, and some are known to contribute to more health problems than others. For example, the *2010 Dietary Guidelines for Americans* recommend that individuals limit their saturated fat intake to no more than 10 percent of their calories because saturated fat has been associated with poor health outcomes (U.S. Department of Agriculture and U.S. Department of Health and Human Services 2010), including cardiovascular disease and stroke. The *Guidelines* also recommend Americans limit their *trans* fat intake as much as possible because of similar poor health associations. Because saturated and *trans* fat intake should be limited, Americans should replace them with monounsaturated and polyunsaturated fats. Sources of these fats tend to have a higher nutritional value and are not associated with the same health consequences.

Among the polyunsaturated fats, omega 3 and omega 6 fatty acids are known as the essential fats. These two fatty acids cannot be synthesized by the body, yet are essential to health. As such, these two polyunsaturated fats must be consumed through the diet. Alpha-linolenic acid (ALA), eicosapentaenoic acid (EPA), and docosahexaenoic acid (DHA) are three of the omega 3 fatty acids, and these omega 3s can be found in fish (e.g., salmon) as well as plant oils (e.g., flaxseed oil). Omega 3 fatty acids have received a lot of attention due to their associations with improving fetal development and reducing inflammation and, as a result, are commonly sold in supplement form. Unlike omega 3 fatty acids, most Americans consume sufficient amounts of omega 6 fatty acids. Linolenic acid, one of the most commonly consumed omega 6 fatty acids, is readily found in meat and dairy products.

Protein

Protein, the third essential macronutrient, is essential for building new body tissue. Similar to the proteins found in the body, dietary proteins are made up of long chains of amino acids, also called polypeptides. There are 20 amino acids that make up these polypeptides. While all amino acids

Table 1.1 The various types of amino acids

Essential amino acids	Nonessential amino acids	Conditionally essential amino acids
Histidine	Alanine	Arginine
Isoleucine	Asparagine	Cysteine
Leucine	Aspartic acid	Glycine
Lysine	Glutamic acid	Glutamine
Methionine	Selenocysteine	Proline
Phenylalanine	Serine	Tyrosine
Threonine		
Tryptophan		
Valine		

are structurally similar, the differentiating characteristic is each amino acid's unique side group.

Amino acids fall into one of three categories: essential, nonessential, and conditionally essential. Essential amino acids are ones that cannot be synthesized in the human body, and therefore, must be ingested through the diet. There are nine essential amino acids, which are listed in Table 1.1. Nonessential amino acids are ones that the body can make in sufficient amounts to meet human needs and, therefore, do not have to be ingested. Conditionally essential amino acids are similar to nonessential amino acids in that they are typically produced in sufficient amounts by the human body; however, under stressful situations, the body may not be able to produce sufficient amounts. Thus, in order to meet the body's demands in times of stress, individuals should consume these amino acids through the diet.

Energy Balance

It is important for patients to keep in mind that their calorie needs may decrease as their body weight decreases (Bray 1969, 397–98; Leibel, Rosenbaum, and Hirsch 1995, 621–28) During the process of weight reduction, patients may need to further decrease their caloric intake or increase their physical activity levels in order to maintain a caloric deficit and continue losing weight. Otherwise the patient's weight may plateau, or stay at one amount, for an extended period of time, causing distress and frustration.

Adipose Tissue

Adipose, or fat, tissue is the primary target for weight management programs because an excessive build-up of this connective tissue is usually what contributes to high weight status and therefore endangers the health of the patients. There are two major types of adipose tissue: brown adipose tissue and white adipose tissue. The brown adipose tissue, primarily found in newborns, functions as a heat generator to keep human beings warm. Its high mitochondrial content gives it a brown appearance (Enerback 2009, 2021–23). On the other hand, the white adipose tissue makes up the majority of fat tissue in human beings, and this tissue primarily functions as energy storage. Energy gets stored as triacylglycerides in white cells called adipocytes. These white cells are what give the white adipose tissue its color.

Adipose tissue will accumulate in various locations throughout the human body. It can be found under the skin (subcutaneous), in and around vital organs and muscles, and even in bone marrow. Regardless of the location, adipose tissue is highly vascular and contains many small blood vessels. These blood vessels deliver nutrients, enzymes, and hormones to and from the adipose tissue. In a fed state, hormones such as insulin will trigger the storage of calories as fat. In a starvation state, hormones such as glucagon will trigger the breakdown of fat tissue, a process known as lipolysis.

When energy is consumed in excess (i.e., positive calorie or energy balance), adipose tissue will grow in one of two ways: by increasing in number or increasing in size (Spalding et al. 2008, 783–87). It has been suggested, however, that the number of adipocytes in the human body is set early in life and that these cells will primarily increase in size when energy intake exceeds energy expended (Spalding et al. 2008, 783–87).

During periods of negative energy balance, the size of adipocytes will decrease as the triacylglycerides within the cells are mobilized and broken down for energy. This decrease in size will ultimately result in weight loss. The number of adipocytes, however, can only be decreased through surgical procedures such as those described in Chapter 11.

Set Point Theory

Just as adult height and shoe size are determined by genetics, an individual's weight is also determined, to some extent, by genetics. For example, an individual's body frame size and musculature are determined by genetics, and these are just two of the factors that will influence weight status. As such, individuals will have a weight at which their body functions optimally, and this weight is commonly known as their set point.

Under the auspices of the set point theory (Harris 1990, 3310–18), the adult human body has a predetermined weight, or set point, at which it prefers to be. In an attempt to keep the body at this weight, an individual's metabolism will fluctuate, causing a reduction in energy expenditure in times of starvation and an increase in expenditure in times of overfeeding. This metabolic fluctuation is thought to have been a survival mechanism of earlier eras, during which human beings had to scavenge for food and were routinely subjected to famine.

A more recent version of the set point theory, known as the settling point theory, has been proposed by some researchers (Farias, Cuevas, and Rodriguez 2011, 85–9). According to this theory, weight is determined by environmental factors (food environment, physical activity environment) in addition to genetics. As such, weight may not change until these environmental factors are altered and made more conducive to a healthier weight status. This theory helps explain the frustrating weight plateaus that some weight loss patients experience while participating in a weight management programs.

When possible, clinicians should explain the set point and settling point theories to their patients before beginning a weight management program. This helps patients mentally prepare for the weight loss plateaus they might experience, and it also helps the patient better understand what body weight is feasible and achievable for him or her.

Summary

In order to manage weight, caloric intake must be balanced with caloric output. It is important for clinicians to recognize how dietary intake influences the caloric intake side of the energy balance equation in order to help patients maintain and lose weight during a comprehensive weight management program.

References

Bray, G. 1969. "Effect of Caloric Restriction on Energy Expenditure in Obese Patients." *The Lancet* 294, no. 7617, pp. 397–98. doi:10.1016/s0140-6736(69)90109-3

Enerback, S. 2009. "The Origins of Brown Adipose Tissue." *The New England Journal of Medicine* 360, no. 19, pp. 2021–23. doi:10.1056/NEJMcibr0809610

Farias, M.M., A.M. Cuevas, and F. Rodriguez. 2011. "Set-Point Theory and Obesity." *Metabolic Syndrome and Related Disorders* 9, no. 2, pp. 85–89. doi:10.1089/met.2010.0090

Harris, R.B. 1990. "Role of Set-Point Theory in Regulation of Body Weight." *FASEB Journal: Official Publication of the Federation of American Societies for Experimental Biology* 4, no. 15, pp. 3310–18. doi:10.1096/fj.1530-6860

Leibel, R.L., M. Rosenbaum, and J. Hirsch. 1995. "Changes in Energy Expenditure Resulting from Altered Body Weight." *New England Journal of Medicine* 332, no. 10, pp. 621–28. doi:10.1056/nejm199503093321001

Spalding, K.L., E. Arner, P.O. Westermark, S. Bernard, B.A. Buchholz, O. Bergmann, L. Blomqvist, J. Hoffstedt, E. Näslund, and T. Britton. 2008. "Dynamics of Fat Cell Turnover in Humans." *Nature* 453, no. 7196, pp. 783–87. doi:10.1038/nature06902

U.S. Department of Agriculture and U.S. Department of Health and Human Services. December 2010. *Dietary Guidelines for Americans, 2010*. 7th ed. Washington, DC: U.S. Government Printing Office.

CHAPTER 2

Epidemiology and Health Consequences of Obesity

The prevalence of overweight and obesity among industrialized nations such as the United States has been increasing over the past several decades. In turn, this has led to higher rates of chronic disease and increased health care costs. Clinicians must understand the epidemiology of overweight and obesity in order to properly articulate the associated risks of these conditions. This chapter will focus on the history of the current American obesity epidemic, its associated health consequences, and how it is impacting the lives of those diagnosed with these conditions.

Obesity Prevalence

In the 1970s, the United States began conducting mass surveillance of Americans' health and nutrition status through the National Health and Nutrition Examination Survey (NHANES) (Centers for Disease Control and Prevention, National Center for Health Statistics 2011). Between 1976 and 1980, NHANES II data estimated that roughly 31.5 percent of American adults were considered overweight (Body Mass Index (BMI) ≥25 but <30) and 14.5 percent were considered obese (BMI ≥30) (Flegal et al. 1998, 39–47).

Throughout the years, however, the percentage of adults classified as overweight has increased slightly, but the percentage classified as obese has more than doubled. Based on the latest NHANES data, ~33 percent of American adults are now considered overweight and an additional 34.9 percent of American adults are considered obese (Ogden et al. 2014, 806–14). In short, these data indicate that the majority of the adult population in the United States is now either overweight or obese, a statistic that warrants the term obesity epidemic.

Over a similar timeframe, an increase in the prevalence of overweight and obese children has also been observed. In NHANES II, 5 percent of U.S. children ages 2 to 19 years were obese (defined as having a BMI-for-age percentile ≥95th percentile); however, the latest NHANES data suggest that roughly 15 percent of children ages 2 to 19 years are overweight and 16.9 percent are obese. In particular, the statistics for adolescents in the age group 12 to 19 years are even more startling. Only 5 percent of adolescents were obese in 1980, but 21 percent were obese in 2011 to 2012 (Ogden et al. 2014, 806–14). This indicates that the number of obese adolescents has more than quadrupled in approximately three decades. Because obese children (as young as 2 years old) are more likely to become obese adults (Freedman et al. 2001, 712–18; Freedman et al. 2005, 22–27; Freedman et al. 2009, 805–11; Guo and Chumlea 1999, 145S–8S), it is imperative to address weight issues and intervene with a comprehensive weight management program as early as possible.

Disparities in Obesity

Although overweight and obesity are two widespread conditions, it is important to recognize that they do not affect all populations equally.

Among race and ethnicity subgroups in the United States, obesity prevalence is higher in minority populations. In 2011–2012, 77.9 percent of Hispanic adults and 76.2 percent of non-Hispanic black adults were considered either overweight or obese, whereas only 67.2 percent of non-Hispanic white adults and 38.6 percent of non-Hispanic Asian adults were overweight or obese (Ogden et al. 2014, 806–14). A similar trend was observed for obesity where 42.5 percent of Hispanic and 47.8 percent of non-Hispanic black adults were obese versus 32.6 percent and 10.8 percent of non-Hispanic white and non-Hispanic Asian adults, respectively, were obese.

Disparities among racial or ethnic groups also exist in children. Among American children in the age group 2 to 19 years, there is a lower prevalence of obesity among non-Hispanic Asian (8.6 percent obese) and non-Hispanic white (14.1 percent) children than among non-Hispanic black (20.2 percent) and Hispanic children (22.4 percent)

(Ogden et al. 2014, 806–14). In addition, obesity is less prevalent among preschoolers (8.4 percent of 2- to 5-year olds are obese) than among school-age children (17.7 percent of 6- to 11-year olds) and adolescents (20.5 percent of 12- to 19-year olds).

In addition to racial or ethnic disparities, there appears to be an association between obesity and an individual's or family's income level. Data from 2005 to 2008 suggest among adult women, the prevalence of obesity increases when the income level decreases (29 percent of high-income adult women are obese versus 42 percent of low-income women) (Ogden et al. 2010, 1–8). This same trend, however, is neither observed among men nor is it observed across the entire adult population. Overall, 41 percent of high-income and 39 percent of middle-income American adults are obese, whereas only 20 percent of low-income adults are obese.

The relationship between the family income level and obesity in school-age children appears to be a bit more complex (Wang and Zhang 2006, 707–16) making inferences between these two variables more difficult to generate. However, the literature does show that low-income preschoolers are more likely to be obese (U.S. Department of Health and Human Services, Centers for Disease Control and Prevention 2014, 1) than their higher-income counterparts. In addition, given the positive association between the income level and education attainment, it should also be noted that the prevalence of obesity among children from well-educated families has been on the decline, whereas obesity among children from less-educated families has continued to increase (Frederick 2014, 1338–42).

Obesity-Related Diseases

Carrying excess body weight and, in particular, excess body fat puts an intense strain on the human body. When this strain persists for years or decades, chronic diseases may develop. The following section will review chronic diseases associated with obesity in both adults and children.

Cardiovascular Disease

Diseases of the cardiovascular system are a leading cause of death in the United States, with coronary heart disease contributing to 611,105 deaths (#1 leading cause of death) and stroke contributing to 128,978 deaths (#5 leading cause of death) in 2013 alone (U.S. Department of Health and Human Services, Centers for Disease Control and Prevention 2015). The hallmarks of cardiovascular disease (CVD) include atherosclerosis, elevated blood lipids, high blood pressure, and elevated inflammatory markers. Not surprisingly, all of the aforementioned hallmarks are also associated with obesity. Approximately 36 percent of obese adults and 26 percent of overweight adults are hypertensive, and ~50 percent of obese adults and 44 percent of overweight adults have dyslipidemia (Saydah et al. 2014, 1888–95).

Overweight children also exhibit many of the hallmarks associated with CVD. One study found that overweight schoolchildren were 2.4 to 7.1 times more likely than their normal weight counterparts to have high total cholesterol, low-density lipoprotein, and triglycerides (Freedman et al. 2005, 22–27). This is important to note because these risk factors will track into adulthood (Bao et al. 1997, 1749–54; Berenson et al. 1998, 1650–56), raising the risk of a CVD event and potentially limiting lifespan and longevity (Daniels 2006, 47–67).

Type 2 Diabetes Mellitus

Type 2 diabetes mellitus (T2DM) is considered a chronic disease because it tends to develop over several years (as opposed to Type 1 diabetes mellitus, an autoimmune disease that develops much more quickly). In T2DM, the body's cells become resistant to insulin, causing the pancreas to overproduce insulin and the blood glucose to rise. Excess body fat contributes to the development of this insulin-resistant state. As such, most patients with T2DM are overweight, and between 50 and 60 percent are clinically obese (Leibson et al. 2001, 1584–89).

T2DM was previously dubbed adult-onset diabetes because the condition was primarily seen in adults. However, because of the rise in childhood obesity, T2DM is now more common in children, thus making the term adult-onset diabetes obsolete. Obesity is one of defining characteristics of T2DM in children (Rosenbloom et al. 2008, 512–26), with the overwhelming majority of new childhood T2DM cases being seen in obese children (Reinehr 2005, S105–10). Although the prevalence of T2DM among children is still low (~0.18 percent), it is higher in children in the age group 10 to 19 years and in African-American children (Pettitt et al. 2014, 402–8). If current trends continue, the number of children with T2DM will quadruple by 2050 (Imperatore et al. 2012, 2515–20).

Intensive weight management programs have shown to slow the development of T2DM. In the Diabetes Prevention Program, researchers demonstrated that a 7 percent weight loss coupled with an intensive lifestyle program could delay the onset of T2DM in adult participants with prediabetes (a condition which precedes a diagnosis of T2DM) (Knowler et al. 2002, 393–403). Similarly, the treatment goals for children and adolescents with T2DM include reducing weight gain while maintaining linear growth and promoting physical activity (Halpern et al. 2010).

Cancer

Cancer is the second leading cause of death in the United States (U.S. Department of Health and Human Services, Centers for Disease Control and Prevention 2015), and both overweight and obesity have been associated with a myriad of cancers.

Breast, endometrial, and prostate cancers are closely linked with weight status. Breast cancer alone was responsible for >41,000 deaths in the United States in 2013, and postmenopausal women who are overweight and obese appear to have a higher risk for developing breast cancer than normal weight women (Vainio and Bianchini 2002; van den Brandt et al. 2000, 514–27). There also appears to be a strong association with between obesity and endometrial cancer in women (Wolk et al. 2001, 13–21). More than 27,000 men died of prostate cancer in 2013, and obesity has been shown to increase risk of high grade (Gong et al. 2006, 1977–83) and aggressive (Allott, Masko, and Freedland 2013, 800–9) prostate cancer.

Colon, colorectal, and rectal cancers, all of which have long been associated with dietary intake, have also been linked to weight status. A 2013 meta-analysis concluded that both general and central obesity were associated with a higher risk of developing colorectal cancer (Ma et al. 2013, e53916). Similarly, higher BMI is associated with colon cancer, but the association appears stronger in men than women (Larsson and Wolk 2007, 556–65).

Further links between obesity and cancer risk are explored on the National Cancer Institute's website (National Institutes of Health, National Cancer Institute 2012).

Other Chronic Illnesses

Although CVD, T2DM, and cancer are three of the major chronic diseases associated with overweight and obesity, there are additional conditions associated with overweight and obesity, which can hinder overall quality of life.

In addition to associating obesity with CVD, T2DM, and cancer, a 2009 systematic review and meta-analysis also found significant associations between obesity in adults and asthma, osteoarthritis, and chronic back pain (Guh et al. 2009, 88). Although these conditions may not be life-threatening alone, they can lead to decreased productivity, performance, and functioning. Fortunately, weight loss appears to improve functioning among those with some forms of osteoarthritis (Christensen, Astrup, and Bliddal 2005, 20–27), and it also improves lung function and related symptoms in obese adults with asthma (Stenius-Aarniala et al. 2000, 827–32).

With all of these chronic diseases being more prevalent among obese individuals than normal weight individuals, it should come as no surprise that longevity and life expectancy is also shorter among obese individuals. It has been estimated that very obese, young adult men lose as much as 8.4 years off their lives as a result of their obesity, and very obese, young adult women losing about the same amount (Grover et al. 2015, 114–22). More importantly, though, is the loss of healthy-life years, or the years an individual was living a healthy life not impacted by disease. The number of healthy-life years lost for obese individuals was up to four times higher the number of life years lost due to obesity. This indicates a significant impairment in quality of life, which could lead to a host of other conditions including mental health impairment.

Mental Health and Obesity

Clinicians will often focus on reducing and controlling the physiological ramifications of obesity, but they should also make sure to identify and treat the psychological consequences as well. The psychological toll of obesity can be high, as obese individuals have been shown to be at higher risk of anxiety, mood, and major depressive disorders than those with a normal or even overweight BMI (Scott et al. 2008, 97–105).

Although a causal mechanism has not yet been fully elucidated in the scientific literature, the relationship between obesity and depression is strong. In some cases, poor mental health may precede the development of obesity, and there is evidence suggesting that children who reported having major depression had a high likelihood of becoming obese as an adult (Pine et al. 2001, 1049–56; Stunkard, Faith, and Allison 2003, 330–37). In other cases, it is posited that obesity may lead to poor mental health later in life, such as in one study that found obese adolescents were nearly two times more likely to develop depression in young adulthood than their nonobese counterparts (Herva et al. 2006, 520–27).

Addiction is another psychological problem that can go hand-in-hand with obesity. Just as individuals can become addicted to nicotine and alcohol, an addiction to food has also been described in the literature (Gearhardt, Corbin, and Brownell 2009, 1–7). Although eating is an innate behavior most often influenced by physiological mechanisms, eating and overeating can also become a coping mechanism for individuals experiencing stress and anxiety. Multiple occasions of overeating coupled with inadequate physical activity (which is often seen with depressed patients) can lead to rapid weight gain and obesity. As such, it is imperative that clinicians screen their patients for potential conditions such as binge eating disorder and night eating disorder to ensure these underlying conditions will not impede weight loss success.

Summary

Over the past several decades, the percentage of American adults and children who are overweight and obese has been on the rise. The health consequences associated with overweight and obesity can have a substantial impact on quality of life, morbidity, and mortality; thus, prevention and early treatment of these conditions should be sought.

References

Allott, E.H., E.M. Masko, and S.J. Freedland. 2013. "Obesity and Prostate Cancer: Weighing the Evidence." *European Urology* 63, no. 5, pp. 800–9. doi:10.1016/j.eururo.2012.11.013

Bao, W., S.R. Srinivasan, R. Valdez, K.J. Greenlund, W.A. Wattigney, and G.S. Berenson. 1997. "Longitudinal Changes in Cardiovascular Risk from Childhood to Young Adulthood in Offspring of Parents with Coronary Artery Disease: The Bogalusa Heart Study." *Jama* 278, no. 21, pp. 1749–54. doi:10.1001/jama.1997.03550210047037

Berenson, G.S., S.R. Srinivasan, W. Bao, W.P. Newman 3rd, R.E. Tracy, and W.A. Wattigney. 1998. "Association Between Multiple Cardiovascular Risk Factors and Atherosclerosis in Children and Young Adults. The Bogalusa Heart Study." *The New England Journal of Medicine* 338, no. 23, pp. 1650–56. doi:10.1056/NEJM199806043382302

Centers for Disease Control and Prevention, National Center for Health Statistics. 2011. "National Health and Nutrition Examination Survey - History." www.cdc.gov/nchs/nhanes/history.htm (accessed June 15, 2015).

Christensen, R., A. Astrup, and H. Bliddal. 2005. "Weight Loss: The Treatment of Choice for Knee Osteoarthritis? A Randomized Trial." *Osteoarthritis and Cartilage* 13, no 1, pp. 20–27. doi:10.1016/j.joca.2004.10.008

Daniels, S.R. 2006. "The Consequences of Childhood Overweight and Obesity." *The Future of Children* 16, no. 1, pp. 47–67. doi:10.1353/foc.2006.0004

Flegal, K.M., M.D. Carroll, R.J. Kuczmarski, and C.L. Johnson. 1998. "Overweight and Obesity in the United States: Prevalence and Trends, 1960–1994." *International Journal of Obesity and Related Metabolic Disorders: Journal of the International Association for the Study of Obesity* 22, no. 1, pp. 39–47. doi:10.1038/sj.ijo.0800541

Frederick, C.B., K. Snellman, and R.D. Putnam. 2014. "Increasing Socioeconomic Disparities in Adolescent Obesity." *Proceedings of the National Academy of Sciences of the United States of America* 111, no. 4, pp. 1338–42. doi:10.1073/pnas.1321355110

Freedman, D.S., L.K. Khan, W.H. Dietz, S.R. Srinivasan, and G.S. Berenson. 2001. "Relationship of Childhood Obesity to Coronary Heart Disease Risk Factors in Adulthood: The Bogalusa Heart Study." *Pediatrics* 108, no. 3, pp. 712–18. doi:10.1542/peds.108.3.712

Freedman, D.S., L.K. Khan, M.K. Serdula, W.H. Dietz, S.R. Srinivasan, and G.S. Berenson. 2005. "The Relation of Childhood BMI to Adult Adiposity: The Bogalusa Heart Study." *Pediatrics* 115, no. 1, pp. 22–27.

Freedman, D.S., J. Wang, J.C. Thornton, Z. Mei, A.B. Sopher, R.N. Pierson Jr, W.H. Dietz, and M. Horlick. 2009. "Classification of Body Fatness by Body Mass Index-for-Age Categories among Children." *Archives of Pediatrics and Adolescent Medicine* 163, no. 9, pp. 805–11. doi:10.1001/archpediatrics.2009.104

Gearhardt, A.N., W.R. Corbin, and K.D. Brownell. 2009. "Food Addiction: An Examination of the Diagnostic Criteria for Dependence." *Journal of Addiction Medicine* 3, no. 1, pp. 1–7. doi:10.1097/ADM.0b013e318193c993

Gong, Z., M.L. Neuhouser, P.J. Goodman, D. Albanes, C. Chi, A.W. Hsing, S.M. Lippman, E.A. Platz, M.N. Pollak, I.M. Thompson, and A.R. Kristal. 2006. "Obesity, Diabetes, and Risk of Prostate Cancer: Results from the Prostate Cancer Prevention Trial." *Cancer Epidemiology, Biomarkers and Prevention: A Publication of the American Association for Cancer Research, Cosponsored by the American Society of Preventive Oncology* 15, no. 10, pp. 1977–83. doi:10.1158/1055-9965.epi-06-0477

Grover, S.A., M. Kaouache, P. Rempel, L. Joseph, M. Dawes, D.C. Lau, and I. Lowensteyn. 2015. "Years of Life Lost and Healthy Life-Years Lost from Diabetes and Cardiovascular Disease in Overweight and Obese People: A Modelling Study." *The Lancet Diabetes and Endocrinology* 3, no. 2, pp. 114–22. doi:10.1016/s2213-8587(14)70229-3

Guo, S.S., and W.C. Chumlea. 1999. "Tracking of Body Mass Index in Children in Relation to Overweight in Adulthood." *The American Journal of Clinical Nutrition* 70, no. 1, pp. 145S–8S.

Guh, D.P., W. Zhang, N. Bansback, Z. Amarsi, C.L. Birmingham, and A.H. Anis. 2009. "The Incidence of Co-Morbidities Related to Obesity and Overweight: A Systematic Review and Meta-Analysis." *BMC Public Health* 9, no. 1, p. 88. doi:10.1186/1471-2458-9-88

Halpern, A., M.C. Mancini, M.E. Magalhaes, M. Fisberg, R. Radominski, M.C. Bertolami, A. Bertolami, M.E. de Melo, M.T. Zanella, M.S. Queiroz, and M. Nery. 2010. "Metabolic Syndrome, Dyslipidemia, Hypertension and Type 2 Diabetes in Youth: From Diagnosis to Treatment." *Diabetology and Metabolic Syndrome* 2, no. 1, p. 55. doi:10.1186/1758-5996-2-55

Herva, A., J. Laitinen, J. Miettunen, J. Veijola, J.T. Karvonen, K. Läksy, and M. Joukamaa. 2006. "Obesity and Depression: Results from the Longitudinal Northern Finland 1966 Birth Cohort Study." *International Journal of Obesity* 30, no. 3, pp. 520–27. doi:10.1038/sj.ijo.0803174

Imperatore, G., J.P. Boyle, T.J. Thompson, D. Case, D. Dabelea, R.F. Hamman, J.M. Lawrence, A.D. Liese, L.L. Liu, E.J. Mayer-Davis, B.L. Rodriguez, and

D. Standiford. 2012. "Projections of Type 1 and Type 2 Diabetes Burden in the U.S. Population Aged <20 Years Through 2050: Dynamic Modeling of Incidence, Mortality, and Population Growth." *Diabetes Care* 35, no. 12, pp. 2515–20. doi:10.2337/dc12-0669

Knowler, W.C., E. Barrett-Connor, S.E. Fowler, R.F. Hamman, J.M. Lachin, E.A. Walker, D.M. Nathan, and Diabetes Prevention Program Research Group. 2002. "Reduction in the Incidence of Type 2 Diabetes with Lifestyle Intervention or Metformin." *The New England Journal of Medicine* 346, no. 6, pp. 393–403. doi:10.1056/NEJMoa012512

Larsson, S.C., and A. Wolk. 2007. "Obesity and Colon and Rectal Cancer Risk: A Meta-Analysis of Prospective Studies." *The American Journal of Clinical Nutrition* 86, no. 3, pp. 556–65.

Leibson, C.L., D.F. Williamson, L.J. Melton 3rd, P.J. Palumbo, S.A. Smith, J.E. Ransom, P.L. Schilling, and K.M. Narayan. 2001. "Temporal Trends in BMI Among Adults with Diabetes." *Diabetes Care* 24, no. 9, pp. 1584–89. doi:10.2337/diacare.24.9.1584

Ma, Y., Y. Yang, F. Wang, P. Zhang, C. Shi, Y. Zou, and H. Qin. 2013. "Obesity and Risk of Colorectal Cancer: A Systematic Review of Prospective Studies." *PloS One* 8, no. 1, e53916. doi:10.1371/journal.pone.0053916

National Institutes of Health, National Cancer Institute. 2012. "Obesity and Cancer Risk." www.cancer.gov/about-cancer/causes-prevention/risk/obesity/obesity-fact-sheet#q6 (accessed June 13, 2015).

Ogden, C.L., M.D. Carroll, B.K. Kit, and K.M. Flegal. 2014. "Prevalence of Childhood and Adult Obesity in the United States, 2011–2012." *Jama* 311, no. 8, pp. 806–14. doi:10.1001/jama.2014.732

Ogden, C.L., M.M. Lamb, M.D. Carroll, and K.M. Flegal. 2010. "Obesity and Socioeconomic Status in Adults: United States, 2005–2008." *NCHS Data Brief* 50, no. 50, pp. 1–8.

Pettitt, D.J., J. Talton, D. Dabelea, J. Divers, G. Imperatore, J.M. Lawrence, A.D. Liese, B. Linder, E.J. Mayer-Davis, C. Pihoker, S.H. Saydah, D.A. Standiford, and R.F. Hamman. 2014. "Prevalence of Diabetes in U.S. Youth in 2009: The SEARCH for Diabetes in Youth Study." *Diabetes Care* 37, no. 2, pp. 402–08. doi:10.2337/dc13-1838

Pine, D.S., R.B. Goldstein, S. Wolk, and M.M. Weissman. 2001. "The Association Between Childhood Depression and Adulthood Body Mass Index." *Pediatrics* 107, no. 5, pp. 1049–56. doi:10.1542/peds.107.5.1049

Reinehr, T. 2005. "Clinical Presentation of Type 2 Diabetes Mellitus in Children and Adolescents." *International Journal of Obesity* 29, pp. S105–10. doi:10.1038/sj.ijo.0803065

Rosenbloom, A.L., J.H. Silverstein, S. Amemiya, P. Zeitler, and G.J. Klingensmith. 2008. "Type 2 Diabetes Mellitus in the Child and Adolescent." *Pediatric Diabetes* 9, no. 5, pp. 512–26. doi:10.1111/j.1399-5448.2008.00429.x

Saydah, S., K.M. Bullard, Y. Cheng, M.K. Ali, E.W. Gregg, L. Geiss, and G. Imperatore. 2014. "Trends in Cardiovascular Disease Risk Factors by Obesity Level in Adults in the United States, NHANES 1999–2010." *Obesity (Silver Spring, Md.)* 22, no. 8, pp. 1888–95. doi:10.1002/oby.20761

Scott, K.M., M.A. McGee, J.E. Wells, and M.A.O. Browne. 2008. "Obesity and Mental Disorders in the Adult General Population." *Journal of Psychosomatic Research* 64, no. 1, pp. 97–105. doi:10.1016/j.jpsychores.2007.09.006

Stenius-Aarniala, B., T. Poussa, J. Kvarnstrom, E.L. Gronlund, M. Ylikahri, and P. Mustajoki. 2000. "Immediate and Long Term Effects of Weight Reduction in Obese People with Asthma: Randomised Controlled Study." *BMJ (Clinical Research Ed.)* 320, no. 7238, pp. 827–32. doi:10.1136/bmj.320.7238.827

Stunkard, A.J., M.S. Faith, and K.C. Allison. 2003. "Depression and Obesity." *Biological Psychiatry* 54, no. 3, pp. 330–37. doi:10.1016/s0006-3223(03)00608-5

U.S. Department of Health and Human Services, Centers for Disease Control and Prevention. 2014. "Childhood Obesity Facts." www.cdc.gov/obesity/data/childhood.html (accessed May 15, 2015).

U.S. Department of Health and Human Services, Centers for Disease Control and Prevention. 2015. "National Center for Health Statistics, Leading Causes of Death." www.cdc.gov/nchs/fastats/leading-causes-of-death.htm (accessed June 10, 2015).

Vainio, H., and F. Bianchini. 2002. *Weight Control and Physical Activity*. Vol. 6 of *IARC Handbooks of Cancer Prevention*. Lyon, France: IARC Press.

van den Brandt, P.A., D. Spiegelman, S.S. Yaun, H.O. Adami, L. Beeson, A.R. Folsom, G. Fraser, R.A. Goldbohm, S. Graham, L. Kushi, J.R. Marshall, A.B. Miller, T. Rohan, S.A. Smith-Warner, F.E. Speizer, W.C. Willett, A. Wolk, and D.J. Hunter. 2000. "Pooled Analysis of Prospective Cohort Studies on Height, Weight, and Breast Cancer Risk." *American Journal of Epidemiology* 152, no. 6, pp. 514–27. doi:10.1093/aje/152.6.514

Wang, Y., and Q. Zhang. 2006. "Are American Children and Adolescents of Low Socioeconomic Status at Increased Risk of Obesity? Changes in the Association Between Overweight and Family Income Between 1971 and 2002." *The American Journal of Clinical Nutrition* 84, no. 4, pp. 707–16.

Wolk, A., G. Gridley, M. Svensson, O. Nyrén, J.K. McLaughlin, J.F. Fraumeni, and H.-O. Adami. 2001. "A Prospective Study of Obesity and Cancer Risk (Sweden)." *Cancer Causes and Control* 12, no. 1, pp. 13–21. doi:10.1023/A:1008995217664

CHAPTER 3

Factors Contributing to Overweight and Obesity

As described in the previous chapter, the epidemic of overweight and obesity has escalated over the past several decades, yet a single cause of obesity has never been elucidated. In reality, there is probably no single cause of this epidemic. Instead, it is widely accepted that the obesity epidemic has arisen from a myriad of contributing factors, including those which originate at the individual, interpersonal, and environmental levels. Using a socioecological model as the guiding framework, this chapter will describe these contributing factors and will explain how these factors relate to the accumulation of excessive weight.

Individual-Level Factors

When designing a weight management program, the intervention should be tailored as much as possible to the patient it targets. As such, it is important to understand the underlying, person-specific factors that have contributed or may contribute to the patient's development of obesity. These individual-level factors will vary from person to person, but in general, there are several key nonmodifiable and modifiable factors to consider.

Non-modifiable Risk Factors

When evaluating the individual-level contributors to obesity, family history and genetics are two of the nonmodifiable risk factors that must be taken into consideration.

Family History

Studies have indicated a link between family history of obesity and obesity among preschoolers (He et al. 2000, 1528–36) and schoolchildren (Moussa et al. 1994, 513–15), and this link appears to be consistent for both overweight children and obese children (Kanciruk, Andrews, and Donnon 2014, 244–56). Interestingly, one study looked at the association between family history of obesity and an individuals' risk of developing obesity over time, and the authors concluded that this association appears to have gotten stronger in more contemporary times, indicating that family history might be a stronger influence now than it was in previous generations (Fox et al. 2014, 919–24). Nonetheless, while an individual's propensity for becoming obese may be influenced by his family history, the extent to which this predisposition is moderated by other factors depends on additional individual and environmental factors.

Genetics

Although very few cases of obesity result from a single gene mutation (Farooqi et al. 2007, 237–47), there are some genetic conditions known to contribute to obesity development. Most of these genetic predispositions are due to mutations in genes for hormones regulating hunger and satiety cues, although there are other mutations in genes that code for metabolic processes that impact weight status.

The first genetic mutation that can contribute to the development of obesity is a mutation in the *ob* gene, a gene that codes for the hormone leptin. Leptin is a fat-derived hormone, or adipokine, which regulates satiety by binding to receptors in the hypothalamus. When an individual consumes excess calories and begins storing more fat tissue, more leptin goes into circulation. These elevated levels of circulating leptin then signal satiety by binding to the hypothalamus. Once this binding occurs, theoretically the individual's appetite and food intake will decrease. This cycle should promote maintenance of weight. However, when there is a mutation in the gene coding for leptin, leptin cannot be produced. This lack of leptin leads to dysregulation of the hunger and satiety cues produced by the hypothalamus. In the absence of a satiety signal, food intake remains high, resulting in excessive weight gain.

Although scientists have concluded that a mutation in the *ob* gene will result in leptin deficiency and obesity, this genetic mutation is rare. Most obese individuals produce more-than-adequate amounts of leptin, and the majority of obese individuals actually have high circulating levels of leptin (Considine et al. 1996, 292–95). However, it appears these individuals exhibit leptin-resistance, a condition in which the hypothalamus does not appropriately respond to these high levels of circulating leptin. In the case of leptin-resistance, the obese individual may have high amount of leptin in the bloodstream but he does not experience the satiation necessary to curb appetite. This, in turn, results in a continuation of overconsumption of calories and further weight gain.

Although leptin is the hormone that regulates satiety, its counterpart, ghrelin, is the hormone that regulates hunger. Ghrelin is a polypeptide hormone secreted by the cells of the gastrointestinal tract. When the body is in an acute, unfed state, the cells release ghrelin into circulation, and the ghrelin binds to receptors in the hypothalamus to induce hunger. Once food is ingested and the stomach is stretched, the cells stop producing ghrelin and hunger subsides.

In some genetic disorders, the circulating levels of ghrelin become altered, resulting in overconsumption of calories and excessive weight gain. This pathway has been proposed as a partial cause of the excessive weight gain associated with Prader–Willi syndrome. Prader–Willi syndrome is a genetic disorder characterized by poor muscle tone and high propensity for hyperphagia. Studies have shown that patients with Prader–Willi syndrome have high levels of circulating ghrelin (Cummings et al. 2002, 643–44). Given ghrelin's role in inducing hunger, the high levels seen in patients with Prader–Willi syndrome are thought to directly contribute to hyperphagia and obesity.

In an obese individual without a genetic disorder, circulating ghrelin tends to be lower than that detected in lean individuals (Tschop et al. 2001, 707–09). In theory, this would indicate that obese individuals should experience weaker hunger cues than their lean counterparts. However, hunger is a complex signal influenced by a myriad of factors besides hormones. Thus, other cues may override the ghrelin signal and cause individuals to consume excessive calories.

There are other genetic predispositions and related disorders that can contribute to weight gain and the development of obesity. For example, polymorphisms of the $\beta 3$-adrenergic receptor gene have been implicated in the development of obesity due to the protein's role in lipolysis and regulation of resting metabolic rate (Clément et al. 1995, 352–54). In addition, a mutation in the *FTO* (fat mass and obesity associated) gene has been associated with obesity in both children and adults (Dina et al. 2007, 724–26). Nonetheless, despite the many links between genetic mutations, genetic predispositions, and obesity, most scientists agree that genetics is not the primary factor in obesity development and that it is more likely obesity results from an interaction between genetics and the environment (Choquet and Meyre 2011, 169–79).

Other nonmodifiable risk factors for obesity include age, gender, and race or ethnicity. Socio-economic status and income level are also factors that may or may not be modifiable and can contribute to obesity.

Modifiable Risk Factors

Because the aforementioned factors (e.g., family history, genetics, age, and race or ethnicity) cannot be modified, the goal of most weight management programs will focus on modifying the individual-level factors that can be changed and that are known determinants of weight status. These factors include nutrition-related knowledge of good dietary principles, attitudes and beliefs towards healthy eating, and current dietary and physical activity-related practices.

Knowledge

The first step in most weight management programs is to ensure that the patient knows what a healthy diet is. This first step is considered a primary goal of any weight management program because increasing the patient's knowledge is an individual-level factor that strongly influences food choices and, in turn, the patient's weight status. While knowledge alone is not sufficient to facilitate changes in eating behavior or weight loss, equipping the patient with the proper knowledge to make healthy choices is a necessary step. For example, a clinician must educate a patient on the correct portion sizes for starches and protein-rich foods, and once the patient has been given this information, then he is equipped with the basic knowledge to properly serve himself the right amounts of food to meet his caloric needs. A clinician can gauge a patient's nutrition knowledge early in the intervention process by asking what he already knows about healthy eating or by giving him a short questionnaire such as the one developed by Feren, Torheim, and Lillegaard (2011). While knowledge of dietary principles is necessary for diet-related behavior change, it is rarely sufficient. As such, clinicians must address other factors discussed in this chapter.

Attitudes and Beliefs

Another individual-level factor that can contribute to the development of obesity is an individual's attitude toward and beliefs about food, nutrition, obesity, and health. Having a positive attitude toward a healthful diet has been associated with better weight status in adults (Acheampong and Haldeman 2013), and it makes sense that having a more positive attitude toward healthy eating would serve as good motivation to make healthier food choices. However, not everyone values a healthy diet the same way clinicians and nutritionists do. Because of this, many weight management interventions aim to improve the patient's attitude toward healthful food choices as a means to improving the overall diet and reducing weight status.

Although an adolescent or adult's attitudes toward food and health are important determinants for his own weight status, parental attitude is an important determinant of a child's weight status. For example, the literature has shown that in some minority populations, parents believe that overweight children are still healthy and that these children "will grow out being overweight" (Trigwell et al. 2014, 179–91). These parental attitudes and beliefs are important to uncover early in the assessment process because children depend on their caretakers to feed them and give them direction. If the caretakers do not feel that the child needs to maintain or lose weight, then the child is less likely to succeed during the weight management program.

At all age levels, there are many nutrition-related attitudes that can influence the development of obesity and potentially determine the success of a weight management program. Other such attitudes and beliefs include those toward:

- Losing weight or maintaining a healthy weight (or achieving the weight target set by the clinician)
- Consuming more fruits and vegetables
- Decreasing fried and other high-calorie foods
- Decreasing consumption of calorie-containing and sugar-sweetened beverages
- Controlling portion sizes and overall caloric intake
- Exercising or being more physically active
- Keeping a food record or food log (paper or electronic)

Clinicians should always gauge a patient's attitude and beliefs early in the intervention process in order to ensure that these are not a barrier to the patient's success. If attitudes and beliefs are not found to be supportive of weight management behaviors, then the clinician should focus on changing these before trying to change the patient's eating behavior.

Diet and Physical Activity-Related Behaviors

As expected, an individual's current diet and physical activity-related behaviors play a huge role in determining an individual's risk for overweight and obesity. In this section, the behaviors related to obesity will be discussed. Assessment of these behaviors is discussed in Chapter 4.

Just as obesity is a complex condition, dietary intake is a complex behavior. Because dietary behaviors tend to interact with one another, it is often difficult to tease apart the actual behaviors that result in energy imbalance and the development of obesity. However, there are several dietary intake patterns that are widely thought to contribute to the development of obesity. These behaviors include:

- Low intakes of fruits (Alinia, Hels, and Tetens 2009, 639–47; Vernarelli et al. 2011, 2204–10) and vegetables (Vernarelli et al. 2011, 2204–10)

- High energy-density diets (Pérez-Escamilla et al. 2012, 671–84)
- Inadequate intake of calcium and dairy products (especially among pediatric patients) (Academy of Nutrition and Dietetics 2007, 11)
- High intakes of calorie-containing (Houchins et al. 2012, 1844–50) and sugar-sweetened (Ludwig, Peterson, and Gortmaker 2001, 505–08; Malik, Schulze, and Hu 2006, 274–88) beverages
- High intakes of total dietary fat (Vernarelli et al. 2011, 2204–10)
- High intakes of added sugars (Dietary Guidelines Advisory Committee 2015; Vernarelli et al. 2011, 2204–10)

Because these aforementioned dietary behaviors are associated with weight gain and obesity, clinicians should advise patients to limit these behaviors as much as possible. Further guidance on specific dietary behaviors is provided in later chapters.

When it comes to the association between obesity and physical activity-related behaviors, there appears to be an inverse relationship, meaning that as physical activity levels increase, the risk of obesity decreases. For this reason, the *Physical Activity Guidelines for Americans* by the U.S. Department of Health and Human Services' recommend adults spend at least 150 minutes each week performing moderate intensity aerobic activity and perform muscle-strengthening activities on at least 2 days a week (U.S. Department of Health and Human Services et al. 2008). The Guidelines recommend that children spend at least 60 minutes each day performing moderate to vigorous intensity physical activity, and they also recommend that children perform bone-strengthening activities and muscle-strengthening activities at least 3 days each week.

In addition to promoting physical activity, time spent in sedentary behaviors (e.g., watching television, playing video games, and using the computer) should be limited in order to maximize energy expenditure. This recommendation is especially important with children. The American Academy of Pediatrics recommends that children under age 2 years have no screen time, and those 2 years and older limit their screen time to no more than 2 hours each day (Strasburger et al. 2013, 958–61). While there are no specific recommendations for adults and screen time, longitudinal research has indicated a link between weight gain and time spent in sedentary activities (Thorp et al. 2011, 207–15); thus adults should limit their sedentary time as much as possible.

Both dietary and physical activity-related behaviors are considered largely modifiable because an individual typically has the ability to change these behaviors and make them more conducive to health. However, it is important to note that there are some cases in which an individual may have more challenges with dietary and activity modifications. For example, an individual with multiple food allergies or intolerances may not be able to eat certain foods, thus making it important to keep his menu free of certain otherwise health-promoting foods and beverages. In addition, some individuals may have limitations on physical activity due to advanced age or mobility. In this case, the clinician should work with a physical therapist or other qualified technician to develop an activity plan that meets the patient's abilities.

Psychological Disturbances

Over the past two decades, there has been an enhanced interest in the link between mental wellbeing and obesity. Multiple studies have shown that obese individuals tend to have abnormally low levels of serotonin (Ericsson, Poston, and Foreyt 1996, 733–43), indicating a potential link between the physiological state observed in depressed individuals and those who are obese. In addition, studies have shown a high frequency of mental disorders such as post-traumatic stress disorder, depression, bipolar disorder, addictions, and bulimia among overweight and obese individuals (Kalarchian et al. 2007, 328–34; Pickering et al. 2007, 998–1009; Yanovski et al. 1993, 1472). Nevertheless, a distinct, causal pathway remains unclear.

What does remain clear is that there are some psychiatric conditions that are known to be closely associated with obesity. One of the most widely known is binge eating disorder (BED). BED is a psychiatric condition in which an individual uncontrollably consumes an abnormally large amount of food in one sitting. Individuals with BED are likely to be obese and commonly exhibit other psychological illnesses such as depression and personality disorders (de Zwaan 2001, S51–55). In addition, when compared with their nondisordered counterparts, individuals who are diagnosed with BED are more likely to have poorer overall physical and mental wellbeing, and lower abilities to properly sense hunger and satiety (Hsu et al. 2002, 1398–403).

The treatment of BED usually involves psychotherapy along with medication intervention (Devlin and Fischer 2005, 27–41). Medication interventions using selective serotonin reuptake inhibitors and anticonvulsants have been shown to be effective in reducing weight as well as reducing binge episodes. Appetite suppressants may also be used to curb hunger and reduce intense food cravings among those with BED. (Further medication interventions for obesity will be discussed in more detail in Chapter 10.) It is important, however, that medication intervention be accompanied by intense psychological counseling and cognitive behavioral therapy, as external triggers (e.g., environmental cues and external stresses) can continue to cause binge episodes even when patients are taking their prescribed medications.

Although certain psychiatric medications may assist with weight loss among binge eaters, not all medications are associated with weight loss. In fact, some commonly prescribed antipsychotics have side effects of increased hunger and weight gain (Allison et al. 1999, 1686–96). Because these medications can put patients at an increased risk of weight gain and obesity, patients taking these medications should be closely monitored for weight changes and should seek weight management guidance when necessary.

Interpersonal Factors

The next level of factors that tend to influence an individual's risk of weight gain and obesity is the interpersonal level.

Social Networks

Scientific literature has strongly suggested social networks can positively and negatively influence an individual's weight status. One explanation for this comes from the presumption that social networks tend to share norms and behaviors, including those related to dietary intake and physical activity. For example, adolescents tend to eat similar foods as their friends. As such, when one adolescent elects to eat fast food, his friend is likely to do the same. This notion is further upheld by findings that overweight adolescents were more likely than their normal weight counterparts to have overweight friends (Valente et al. 2009, 202–04).

These shared behaviors and shared norms are deeply engrained in social groups. As such, when attempting to modify the behaviors (i.e., dietary intake) of one individual within the social network, it typically behooves that individual to seek social support from another member of his network. If the individual seeking weight management is a child, this social support should ideally come from a caretaker (e.g., parent, primary guardian) (Gerald et al. 1994, 145–63).

Cultural Factors

Because the United States is a melting pot of individuals from all over the world, clinicians should be prepared to discuss weight management in a culturally appropriate context. Many first-generation immigrants may still follow a non-Western lifestyle, even while living in the United States, and the clinician should be aware of how that particular lifestyle impacts behaviors related to food intake and physical activity.

For clinicians, addressing the cultural factors related to dietary intake and obesity can be a challenging task simply because culture is usually engrained and is difficult to modify. However, it is imperative that clinicians recognize the cultural aspects of a patient's life that can influence his weight status and discuss those aspects as part of the comprehensive weight management program.

A patient's culture or background will often provide insight into dietary behaviors and usual food and nutrient intake. For example, a patient who follows a typical Mexican diet may have higher intakes of corn tortillas and beans than a patient who follows a traditional Asian diet that is high in white rice and colorful vegetables. The traditional diets of many countries and regions around the world tend to be extremely healthful given they contain a variety of unprocessed foods. As such, it is often prudent of the clinician to discuss cultural food habits with the patient as a means of motivating the patient to eat more healthfully.

Like dietary behaviors, physical activity-related behaviors, which also contribute to weight status, can be influenced by the patient's culture. Individuals from non-Westernized countries tend to spend more time being physically active, and this is proposed to contribute to their lower rates of overweight and obesity. Just as clinicians should inquire about a patient's cultural food habits, they should also discuss cultural habits related to physical activity.

As mentioned, individuals living in the United States can be from anywhere around the world; however, after living in the United States for an extended period of time, many people will adapt to the Western lifestyle. This process, dubbed acculturation, may be beneficial in some aspects, but acculturation and the adoption of a more Westernized diet has been associated with weight gain and obesity in some migrant groups (Garcia et al. 2012, 58–64; Nguyen et al. 2015, 389–99). As such, a focus of weight management programs may be on helping a patient to maintain a more traditional diet that is less Westernized and more similar to what his ancestors consumed.

Environmental Factors

Although a patient may be motivated to eat healthy and be physically active, he will be hard-pressed to do so unless the environment in which he lives is conducive to these behaviors. As such, clinicians must also consider the impacts of environmental factors when developing a comprehensive weight management program.

Food and Physical Activity Environments

Food and physical activity environments have been implicated as contributors to the obesity epidemic (Sallis and Glanz 2009, 123–54). Over the past several decades, the physical landscape of most U.S. cities and towns has changed dramatically, and as a result, more people are now living in urbanized areas where healthy foods are less available than convenience foods, and where safe recreational spaces are often limited. These unhealthy environments are conducive to poor dietary intake and a sedentary lifestyle, both of which are correlated with weight gain and obesity.

Although the following list is not exhaustive, it includes many characteristics of food and physical activity environments that may help protect against weight gain and the development of obesity:

- Easily accessible full-scale grocery stores and farmers markets
- Easily accessible food banks and other food assistance programs
- Availability of high-quality produce and healthy foods in grocery and convenience stores, restaurants, and food banks
- Availability of affordable produce and healthy foods in all food establishments
- Easily accessible and safe walking paths, bike trails, and other paths for active transportation
- Availability of recreational facilities and organized sports teams or leagues

Workplaces and Schools

Adults and children spend a good amount of their waking hours at the workplace and at school, respectively. As a result, the food and physical activity environments of these locations are considered to be potential contributors to the obesity epidemic.

Although work schedules and work days will vary from person to person, many adults will spend 40 or more hours each week in the workplace. At the workplace, adults will typically consume at least one meal (although individuals who work longer schedules may eat two or three meals while in the workplace). Because of the enormous amount of time spent by adults in this location, the food environment of the workplace has been implicated as a contributor to adults' dietary habits.

Similar to the large amount of time spent by adults in the workplace, children spend a large amount of time in the school setting. Although some children will only eat one meal at school, others will eat breakfast, lunch, and snacks in this setting. In most schools, children have the option to bring their own foods or purchase foods at the school. For those who purchase food at the school (and for those children who receive free meals), their intake is completely dependent on the types and quantities of food available in the school.

Over the past several decades, organizations and government agencies have been instituting food-related policies to ensure the foods available in workplaces and schools are conducive to health. These kinds of policies and interventions have been widely supported (Dietary Guidelines Advisory Committee 2015) as they have been posited to help promote a healthier weight status among adults and children.

Summary

There are a wide variety of individual, interpersonal, and environmental factors that may play a role in the development of obesity. When counseling patients on techniques for weight management, all of these factors should be carefully examined. In the ensuing chapters, strategies to modify these factors will be discussed.

References

Academy of Nutrition and Dietetics. 2007. "Pediatric Weight Management: Executive Summary of Recommendations." www.andeal.org/topic.cfm?menu=5296&cat=3013 (accessed June, 2015).

Acheampong, I., and L. Haldeman. 2013. "Are Nutrition Knowledge, Attitudes, and Beliefs Associated with Obesity among Low-Income Hispanic and African American Women Caretakers?" *Journal of Obesity* 2013, pp. 1–8. doi:10.1155/2013/123901

Alinia, S., O. Hels, and I. Tetens. 2009. "The Potential Association Between Fruit Intake and Body Weight–A Review." *Obesity Reviews* 10, no. 6, pp. 639–47. doi:10.1111/j.1467-789x.2009.00582.x

Allison, D.B., J.L Mentore, M. Heo, L.P. Chandler, J.C. Cappelleri, M.C. Infante, and P.J. Weiden. 1999. "Antipsychotic-Induced Weight Gain: A Comprehensive Research Synthesis." *American Journal of Psychiatry* 156, no. 11, pp. 1686–96.

Choquet, H., and D. Meyre. 2011. "Genetics of Obesity: What Have We Learned?" *Current Genomics* 12, no. 3, pp. 169–79. doi:10.2174/138920211795677895

Clément, K., C. Vaisse, B.S.J. Manning, A. Basdevant, B. Guy-Grand, J. Ruiz, K.D. Silver, A.R. Shuldiner, P. Froguel, and A.D. Strosberg. 1995. "Genetic Variation in the β3-Adrenergic Receptor and an Increased Capacity to Gain Weight in Patients with Morbid Obesity." *New England Journal of Medicine* 333, no. 6, pp. 352–54. doi:10.1056/nejm199508103330605

Considine, R.V., M.K. Sinha, M.L. Heiman, A. Kriauciunas, T.W. Stephens, M.R. Nyce, J.P. Ohannesian, C.C. Marco, L.J. McKee, T.L. Bauer, and J.F. Caro. 1996. "Serum Immunoreactive-Leptin Concentrations in Normal-Weight and Obese Humans." *New England Journal of Medicine* 334, no. 5, pp. 292–95. doi:10.1056/nejm199602013340503

Cummings, D.E., K. Clement, J.Q. Purnell, C. Vaisse, K.E. Foster, R.S. Frayo, M.W. Schwartz, A. Basdevant, and D.S. Weigle. 2002. "Elevated Plasma Ghrelin Levels in Prader–Willi Syndrome." *Nature Medicine* 8, no. 7, pp. 643–44. doi:10.1038/nm0702-643

de Zwaan, M. 2001. "Binge Eating Disorder and Obesity." *International Journal of Obesity and Related Metabolic Disorders: Journal of the International Association for the Study of Obesity* 25, Suppl 1, pp. S51–55.

Devlin, M.J., and S.E. Fischer. 2005. "Treatment of Binge Eating Disorder." Part 1 of *Eating Disorders Review,* 27–41. Abingdon, UK: Radcliffe.

Dietary Guidelines Advisory Committee. 2015. Scientific Report of the 2015 Dietary Guidelines Advisory Committee. Washington, DC: USDA and U.S. Department of Health and Human Services.

Dina, C., D. Meyre, S. Gallina, E. Durand, A. Körner, P. Jacobson, L.M.S. Carlsson, W. Kiess, V. Vatin, and C. Lecoeur, J. Delplanque, E. Vaillant, F. Pattou, J. Ruiz, J. Weill, C. Levy-Marchal, F. Horber, N. Potoczna, S. Hercberg, C.L. Stunff, P. Bougnères, P. Kovacs, M. Marre, B. Balkau, S. Cauchi, J.-C. Chèvre, and P. Froguel. 2007. "Variation in FTO Contributes to Childhood Obesity and Severe Adult Obesity." *Nature Genetics* 39, no. 6, pp. 724–26. doi:10.1038/ng2048

Ericsson, M., W.S.C. Poston, and J.P. Foreyt. 1996. "Common Biological Pathways in Eating Disorders and Obesity." *Addictive Behaviors* 21, no. 6, pp. 733–43. doi:10.1016/0306-4603(96)00032-9

Farooqi, I.S., T. Wangensteen, S. Collins, W. Kimber, G. Matarese, J.M. Keogh, E. Lank, B. Bottomley, J.L. Fernandez, and I. Ferraz-Amaro. M.T. Dattani, O. Ercan, A.G. Myhre, L. Retterstol, R. Stanhope, J.A. Edge, S. McKenzie, N. Lessan, M. Ghodsi, V. De Rosa, F. Perna, S. Fontana, I. Barroso, D.E. Undlien, and S. O'Rahilly. 2007. "Clinical and Molecular Genetic Spectrum of Congenital Deficiency of the Leptin Receptor." *New England Journal of Medicine* 356, no. 3, pp. 237–47. doi:10.1056/nejmoa063988

Feren, A., L.E. Torheim, and I.T. Lillegaard. 2011. "Development of a Nutrition Knowledge Questionnaire for Obese Adults." *Food and Nutrition Research* 55. doi:10.3402/fnr.v55i0.7271

Fox, C.S., M.J. Pencina, N.L. Heard-Costa, P. Shrader, C. Jaquish, C.J. O'Donnell, R.S. Vasan, L.A. Cupples, and R.B. D'Agostino. 2014. "Trends in the Association of Parental History of Obesity Over 60 Years." *Obesity* 22, no. 3, pp. 919–24. doi:10.1002/oby.20564

Garcia, L., E.B. Gold, L. Wang, X. Yang, M. Mao, and A.V. Schwartz. 2012. "The Relation of Acculturation to Overweight, Obesity, Pre-Diabetes and Diabetes Among U.S. Mexican-American Women and Men." *Ethnicity and Disease* 22, no. 1, pp. 58–64.

Gerald, L.B., A. Anderson, G.D. Johnson, C. Hoff, and R.F. Trimm. 1994. "Social Class, Social Support and Obesity Risk in Children." *Child: Care, Health and Development* 20, no. 3, pp. 145–63. doi:10.1111/j.1365-2214.1994.tb00377.x

He, Q., Z.Y. Ding, D.Y. Fong, and J. Karlberg. 2000. "Risk Factors of Obesity in Preschool Children in China: A Population-Based Case--Control Study." *International Journal of Obesity and Related Metabolic Disorders: Journal of the International Association for the Study of Obesity* 24, no. 11, pp. 1528–36. doi:10.1038/sj.ijo.0801394

Houchins, J.A., J.R. Burgess, W.W. Campbell, J.R. Daniel, M.G. Ferruzzi, G.P. McCabe, and R.D. Mattes. 2012. "Beverage vs. Solid Fruits and Vegetables: Effects on Energy Intake and Body Weight." *Obesity* 20, no. 9, pp. 1844–50. doi:10.1038/oby.2011.192

Hsu, L.K., B. Mulliken, B. McDonagh, D.S. Krupa, W. Rand, C.G. Fairburn, B. Rolls, M.A. McCrory, E. Saltzman, S. Shikora, J. Dwyer, and S. Roberts. 2002. "Binge Eating Disorder in Extreme Obesity." *International Journal of Obesity and Related Metabolic Disorders: Journal of the International Association for the Study of Obesity* 26, no. 10, pp. 1398–403. doi:10.1038/sj.ijo.0802081

Kalarchian, M.A., M.D. Marcus, M.D. Levine, A.P. Courcoulas, P.A. Pilkonis, R.M. Ringham, J.N. Soulakova, L.A. Weissfeld, and D.L. Rofey. 2007. "Psychiatric Disorders among Bariatric Surgery Candidates: Relationship to Obesity and Functional Health Status." *The American Journal of Psychiatry* 164, no. 2, pp. 328–34. doi:10.1176/appi.ajp.164.2.328

Kanciruk, M., J.J.W. Andrews, and T. Donnon. 2014. "Family History of Obesity and Risk of Childhood Overweight and Obesity: A Meta-Analysis." *International Journal of Medical, Health, Pharmaceutical, Biomedical, Engineering* 8, no. 5, pp. 244–56. www.waset.org/publications/9998332

Ludwig, D.S., K.E. Peterson, and S.L. Gortmaker. 2001. "Relation Between Consumption of Sugar-Sweetened Drinks and Childhood Obesity: A Prospective, Observational Analysis." *The Lancet* 357, no. 9255, pp. 505–08. doi:10.1016/s0140-6736(00)04041-1

Malik, V.S., M.B. Schulze, and F.B. Hu. 2006. "Intake of Sugar-Sweetened Beverages and Weight Gain: A Systematic Review." *The American Journal of Clinical Nutrition* 84, no. 2, pp. 274–88.

Moussa, M.A., M.B. Skaik, S.B. Selwanes, O.Y. Yaghy, and S.A. Bin-Othman. 1994. "Factors Associated with Obesity in School Children." *International Journal of Obesity and Related Metabolic Disorders: Journal of the International Association for the Study of Obesity* 18, no. 7, pp. 513–15.

Nguyen, H.H.D., C. Smith, G.L. Reynolds, and B. Freshman. 2015. "The Effect of Acculturation on Obesity Among Foreign-Born Asians Residing in the United States." *Journal of Immigrant and Minority Health* 17, no. 2, pp. 389–99. doi:10.1007/s10903-014-0027-6

Pérez-Escamilla, R., J.E. Obbagy, J.M. Altman, E.V. Essery, M.M. McGrane, Y.P. Wong, J.M. Spahn, and C.L. Williams. 2012. "Dietary Energy Density and Body Weight in Adults and Children: A Systematic Review." *Journal of the Academy of Nutrition and Dietetics* 112, no. 5, pp. 671–84. doi:10.1016/j.jand.2012.01.020

Pickering, R.P., B.F. Grant, S.P. Chou, and W.M. Compton. 2007. "Are Overweight, Obesity, and Extreme Obesity Associated with Psychopathology? Results from the National Epidemiologic Survey on Alcohol and Related Conditions." *The Journal of Clinical Psychiatry* 68, no. 7, pp. 998–1009. doi:10.4088/jcp.v68n0704

Sallis, J.F., and K. Glanz. 2009. "Physical Activity and Food Environments: Solutions to the Obesity Epidemic." *Milbank Quarterly* 87, no. 1, pp. 123–54. doi:10.1111/j.1468-0009.2009.00550.x

Strasburger, V.C., M.J. Hogan, D.A. Mulligan, N. Ameenuddin, D.A. Christakis, C. Cross, D.B. Fagbuyi, D.L. Hill, A. Estin Levine, and C. McCarthy. 2013. "Children, Adolescents, and the Media." *Pediatrics* 132, no. 5, pp. 958–61. doi:10.1542/peds.2013-2656

Thorp, A.A., N. Owen, M. Neuhaus, and D.W. Dunstan. 2011. "Sedentary Behaviors and Subsequent Health Outcomes in Adults: A Systematic Review of Longitudinal Studies, 1996–2011." *American Journal of Preventive Medicine* 41, no. 2, pp. 207–15. doi:10.1016/j.amepre.2011.05.004

Trigwell, J., P.M. Watson, R.C. Murphy, G. Stratton, and N.T. Cable. 2014. "Ethnic Differences in Parental Attitudes and Beliefs About Being Overweight in Childhood." *Health Education Journal* 73, no. 2, pp. 179–91. doi:10.1177/0017896912471035

Tschop, M., C. Weyer, P.A. Tataranni, V. Devanarayan, E. Ravussin, and M.L. Heiman. 2001. "Circulating Ghrelin Levels Are Decreased in Human Obesity." *Diabetes* 50, no. 4, pp. 707–09. doi:10.2337/diabetes.50.4.707

U.S. Department of Health and Human Services, Office of Disease Prevention and Health Promotion. 2008. "Physical Activity Guidelines for Americans." Washington, DC: HHS.

Valente, T.W., K. Fujimoto, C.-P. Chou, and D. Spruijt-Metz. 2009. "Adolescent Affiliations and Adiposity: A Social Network Analysis of Friendships and Obesity." *Journal of Adolescent Health* 45, no. 2, pp. 202–04. doi:10.1016/j.jadohealth.2009.01.007

Vernarelli, J.A., D.C. Mitchell, T.J. Hartman, and B.J. Rolls. 2011. "Dietary Energy Density Is Associated with Body Weight Status and Vegetable Intake in U.S. Children." *The Journal of Nutrition* 141, no. 12, pp. 2204–10. doi:10.3945/jn.111.146092

Yanovski, S.Z., J.E. Nelson, B.K. Dubbert, and R.L. Spitzer. 1993. "Association of Binge Eating Disorder and Psychiatric Comorbidity in Obese Subjects." *The American Journal of Psychiatry* 150, no. 10, pp. 1472–79. doi:10.1176/ajp.150.10.1472

CHAPTER 4

Nutrition Assessment

The first step in the nutritional management of a patient seeking weight guidance is a full nutrition assessment. Nutrition assessment typically involves the evaluation of anthropometric measurements, biochemical data, and physical signs and symptoms, as well as a thorough interview with the patient. This chapter will review each of these aspects of nutrition assessment and explain how they can inform the rest of the weight management program.

Anthropometric Measurements

Anthropometric measurements, or anthropometrics, are physical measurements of the body. They include measurements commonly obtained in clinical settings, such as height and weight, as well as other measurements, such as percent body fat, that require more sophisticated equipment. Because weight by itself is an anthropometric measurement and because a clinical diagnosis of overweight and obesity is typically based on weight and body fat-related proxies, this section will focus on anthropometric measurements of body mass index (BMI), waist circumference, and body fat.

Assessing Body Mass Index

A patient's weight status can be obtained using a number of clinical procedures. One of the most common procedures of the calculation is BMI. In most individuals, BMI is associated with body fatness (Freedman, Horlick, and Berenson 2013, 1417–24; Garrow and Webster 1985, 147–53; Wohlfahrt-Veje et al. 2014, 664–70), thus making a higher BMI more indicative of overweight and obesity. There are several limitations to BMI interpretation, and these limitations will be discussed in more detail later in this section. According to the Academy of Nutrition and

Dietetics, BMI should be obtained (at least) annually in order to detect changes in weight status (Academy of Nutrition and Dietetics 2014).

BMI is relatively easy to obtain as it is calculated from two noninvasive measurements: a patient's height (measured in meters) and weight (measured in kilograms). Prior to obtaining these measurements, it is imperative that clinicians be trained (and periodically retrained) to follow strict, uniform procedures when obtaining a patient's height and weight. Doing so will ensure accuracy of measurements and validity of the resulting weight assessments. Although some hospitals or clinics may write their own protocols, it is highly recommended that the protocols for gathering height and weight measurements be based on gold standard procedures, such as those used in large health assessment studies (e.g., National Health and Nutrition Examination Survey [U.S. Department of Health and Human Services, Centers for Disease Control and Prevention 2013], WHO Multicentre Growth Reference Study [de Onis 2006]).

The procedure by which height, or stature, is obtained depends on the age and physical disposition of the patient, as well as the equipment available to make this assessment. For adults who are able to stand without assistance, a calibrated stadiometer should be used to obtain a standing height measurement. When obtaining this measurement, the clinician should instruct the adult to take off any headwear or footwear prior to stepping onto the stadiometer. Once standing on the stadiometer, the clinician should instruct the adult to face away from the backboard, stand with his feet together and toes slightly apart, and distribute his weight evenly between both feet. When possible, the adult's heels, buttocks, shoulder blades, and head should lightly touch the stadiometer's backboard; however, if this is not possible due to conditions such as kyphosis or obesity, the clinician should ensure the adult's legs are straight and his trunk is vertical. Once the adult's head is in the Frankfort horizontal plane (i.e., the imaginary horizon line from the ear canal to the lower border of the eye orbit is parallel to the ground), the clinician should lower the headpiece onto the adult's head. The clinician should instruct the adult to inhale and stand as tall as possible, and then the measurement should be recorded to the nearest millimeter. When possible, a second measurement using the same procedure should be obtained to ensure accuracy.

The aforementioned procedure can also be used to assess standing height for children 2 years and older who are able to follow the procedure's instructions. However, for children up to 3 years (Beker 2006, 196–97; discussion 197–98) who are unable to follow these instructions or for infants who cannot stand, recumbent length should be used. Recumbent length requires the use of an infantometer, or inflexible length board. Just as with the previous procedure, all headwear and footwear should first be removed. The clinician should place the child supine on the infantometer, positioning the crown of the child's head against the headpiece. The child's legs should be fully extended and feet should be flexed perpendicular to the board's base. The measurement should be captured by placing the foot piece against the feet of the child. Again, a second measurement using the same procedure should be obtained to ensure accuracy of the original measurement. Both measurements should be made to the nearest millimeter.

When measuring recumbent length on young children, it is often difficult to obtain reliable measures. As such, it is recommended to have two clinicians when taking this measurement. One clinician serves to stabilize the child by placing his hands over the child's ears and ensuring the child's head is against the headpiece. The second clinician straightens the child's legs and records the length measurement.

It is important to note that recumbent length and standing height cannot be used interchangeably on children's growth charts. When a recumbent length measurement is being used in lieu of standing height on a children's growth chart, 1 to 2 cm should be added to the recumbent length measurement (Roche and Davila 1974, 313–20; WHO 1995).

For patients who are unable to stand due to musculo-skeletal deformities or other medical conditions, proxy measures can be used to estimate vertical height. Knee height (Chumlea, Guo, and Steinbaugh 1994, 1385–91; Chumlea, Roche, and Steinbaugh 1985, 116–20), upper arm and lower leg length (Stallings and Zemel 1996, 62), and arm span (Jarzem and Gledhill 1993, 761–65; Steele and Chenier 1990, 533–41) are all anthropometric measurements that can be used in conjunction with predictive equations to estimate height. However, when possible, standing height and recumbent length are the preferred procedures.

In addition to height, weight is the second component of BMI. Like height measurements, weight measurements should only be obtained by clinicians who have been adequately trained in the proper procedures. The procedures for obtaining weight measurements should always start with calibrating the scale because this step ensures accuracy of the measurement. Most scales will come with directions as to how to perform a suitable calibration; however, in most cases, a scale can be calibrated by confirming a readout of "0.0 kg" when there is nothing on the weighing platform. When a scale is being calibrated and when it is taking measurement, it is imperative that scales be placed on a hard surface (e.g., tile floor) and not on a soft surface (e.g., carpet floor).

After calibrating the scale but prior to obtaining a weight measurement, the clinician should ensure that the patient is wearing minimal clothing. In an ideal situation, the patient would only wear an examination gown and underpants when getting his weight taken; however, given that weights are often obtained before a patient has the opportunity to change into an examination gown, the clinician should at least ask the patient to remove all outer clothing (e.g., jacket, sweatshirt, hoodie), heavy accessories (e.g., large necklaces, belt), footwear, and headwear.

When using a balance beam or any other scale that requires the patient to be in a standing position, the clinician should direct the patient to stand in the center of the weighing platform, facing toward the clinician. The patient should place his arms to his side and look straight ahead. Once the patient is stable and not moving, the clinician should record the measurement to the nearest 0.1 kg. A repeat measure should then be taken to ensure reliability of the original measurement.

For children under 2 years who are unable to stand or stand still while having their weight taken, weight measurements can be obtained using two alternative methods. First, a pediatric pan scale, or baby scale, can be used. In this procedure, a clinician places the infant or toddler completely in the scale and distributes the child's body weight as evenly as possible across the scale. When the child is still, a measurement is then taken to the nearest 0.001 kg. The second method for obtaining a young child's weight requires an adult to hold the child while having the adult's weight taken on a standing scale. The adult then puts the child down and has his weight taken again. The difference between the adult's weight while holding the child and while not holding the child is calculated, and this measurement is assumed to be the child's actual weight.

For morbidly obese individuals and individuals who are unable to stand, modified scales can be used to gather weight measurements. Most inpatient and long-term care facilities are now equipped with bed scales, which allow weight measurements to be obtained on patients who cannot walk and are bedridden. Wheelchair scales are also commonly available in hospitals and clinics, and these scales can be used to measure the weight status of individuals who cannot walk and are wheelchair-bound. Regardless of what scale is being used, patients should still be encouraged to remove as much clothing as possible prior to having their weight taken. In addition, if a bed or wheelchair scale is being used, any heaving pads, blankets, or other equipment should be removed prior to the weight being taken.

Once a patient's height and weight have been obtained, BMI can be calculated using the formula:

Weight (kg)/Height (m^2). For adults (over 20 years), an individual's BMI can be categorized as follows (National Heart Lung and Blood Institute 1998):

Underweight: BMI < 18.5
Normal weight: BMI ≥ 18.5 but <25
Overweight: BMI ≥ 25 but <30
Obese: BMI ≥ 30

For those adult patients whose BMI ≥ 30, the extent of their obesity can be further posited using the following classifications:

Obesity – Class I: BMI ≥ 30 but <35
Obesity – Class II: BMI ≥ 35 but <40
Obesity – Class III (extreme obesity): BMI ≥ 40

For adult patients who are obese, their class of obesity (in addition to other factors) is often used when determining eligibility for bariatric surgery (Mechanick et al. 2013, S1–27) (please see Chapter 11 for more information on weight loss surgery).

When classifying the BMI of children ages 2 to 19 years, BMI should be plotted on a growth chart in relation to the child's age. To do this, the Centers for Disease Control and Prevention (CDC) recommends clinicians use the gender-specific CDC Growth Charts for children 2 to 19 years (U.S. Department of Health and Human Services, Centers for Disease Control and Prevention, National Center for Health Statistics 2010a). Although there are a number of different CDC Growth Charts, the BMI-for-age chart allows clinicians to plot a child's BMI against his age and determine the child's BMI-for-age percentile. The percentile is then classified as follows (Barlow 2007):

Underweight: BMI percentile less than the 5th percentile
Healthy weight: BMI percentile at or above the 5th percentile but less than the 85th percentile
Overweight: BMI percentile at or above the 85th percentile but less than the 95th percentile
Obesity: BMI percentile at or above the 95th percentile

Children should have their heights and weights measured and their BMI-for-age percentiles calculated at least once every year (Barlow 2007). This will allow clinicians to monitor and track any abnormal changes in BMI-for-age percentiles and will allow for early identification of overweight or obesity.

Children who are 0 to 2 years should have their recumbent length and weight documented using the WHO Growth Charts (U.S. Department of Health and Human Services, Centers for Disease Control and Prevention, National Center for Health Statistics 2010b). Like the CDC Growth Charts, the WHO Growth Charts are gender-specific, but unlike the CDC Charts, the WHO Charts do not track BMI-for-age. Instead, the WHO Charts plot weight against length in these young children and generate a corresponding weight-for-length percentile. There are no cutoff values for overweight or obesity in these young children; however, infants with a percentile below the 2nd percentile and above the 98th percentile are considered have abnormal growth (de Onis 2006) (i.e., less than the 2nd percentile is consider low weight-for-length, and above the 98th percentile is considered high weight-for-length).

When assessing a patient's weight status, most clinicians will use BMI (or BMI-for-age percentiles in children) to guide their evaluation. However, despite the association between BMI and body fatness, BMI should not be used alone to determine an individual's weight status and risk of chronic disease. BMI does not account for other factors, which may impact an individual's body fatness (e.g., age, gender, and lean body mass), nor does it account for the location of fat deposits (e.g., visceral versus central adiposity), which can also impact disease risk. As such, it is recommended that when assessing an adult patient's weight status, the clinician should also include additional anthropometric measurements, such as waist circumference.

Assessing Waist Circumference

In addition to BMI, waist circumference is another anthropometric measurement, which can be used as an indicator of body fatness and weight status in adults (Flegal et al. 2009, 500–508). In particular, a high waist circumference indicates central adiposity, or a condition when fat tissue becomes concentrated in the trunk region. When a patient has a large portion of fat tissue deposited in the central abdominal region, this is known as android obesity. Conversely, when a patient has more of his fat tissue concentrated in the extremities and hips, this is known as gynoid obesity. Android obesity is of clinical significance given the association between this central adiposity (as measured by high waist circumference) and elevated risk of cardiovascular disease, type 2 diabetes, hypercholesterolemia, and hypertension (Chan et al. 1994, 961–69).

Like BMI, waist circumference is a relatively inexpensive, noninvasive measurement to obtain in the clinical setting. The only equipment needed to obtain this measurement is nonstretch measuring tape and a cosmetic pencil. There are multiple procedures for obtaining waist circumference measurements (U.S. Department of Health and Human Services, Centers for Disease Control and Prevention 2013; WHO 2008, 8–11). In the procedure recommended by CDC, the patient should be standing with his arms crossed and his hands on opposite shoulders. The clinician should begin by marking the measurement starting site, the upper lateral border of the right ilium, using the pencil. The measuring tape should then be extended around the patient's full waist, keeping the tape in a horizontal plane parallel to the floor and aligned with the original mark. The tape should be snug, but not pulled to the point it is constricting. Measurements should be recorded to the nearest 0.1 cm and, when possible, repeated for reliability purposes.

Waist circumference recommendations vary based on the gender. The recommended waist circumference for adult women is ≤88 cm (or ≤35 in.) and for adult men is ≤102 cm (or ≤40 in.) (National Heart Lung and Blood Institute 1998). When combined with BMI, waist circumference measurements can help predict disease risk as seen in Table 4.1.

Studies have investigated the use of measurements that account for waist circumference (e.g., waist-to-hip ratios [Czernichow et al. 2011, 680–87; de Koning et al. 2007, 850–56]) and waist-to-stature ratios (Flegal et al. 2009, 500–508) as additional indicators of disease risk and

Table 4.1 Associations between disease risk, adult BMI, and adult waist circumference

	Disease (HTN, T2DM, CVD) risk compared to adults with normal weight and waist circumference	
BMI category (BMI range)	**Men with normal waist circumference (≤102 cm or 40 in.) and women with normal waist circumference (≤88 cm or 35 in.)**	**Men with high waist circumference (>102 cm or 40 in.) and women with high waist circumference (>88 cm or 35 in.)**
Underweight (<18.5)	—	—
Normal weight (18.5–24.9)	—	—
Overweight (25–29.9)	Increased	High
Obesity Class I (30–34.9)	High	Very high
Obesity Class II (35–39.9)	Very high	Very high
Obesity Class III (≥40)	Extremely high	Extremely high

HTN, hypertension; T2DM, Type 2 diabetes mellitus; CVD, cardiovascular disease

Source: Adapted from National Heart Lung and Blood Institute (1998).

weight status. For example, nearly three decades ago, it was posited that a waist-to-hip circumference ratio of >1 for men and >0.85 for women indicated excess accumulation of abdominal fat (Bjorntorp 1987). However, to date, no standards or reference values for these ratios have been widely accepted; thus these ratios are not routinely used in clinical practice.

Most of the links between waist circumference, body fatness, and disease risk have been explored in adult populations. It should be noted, though, some studies have found correlations between waist circumference and cardiovascular risk factors in children (Lee et al. 2006, 188–94; Maffeis et al. 2001, 179–87; Savva et al. 2000, 1453–58). In addition, reference data for waist circumference in children has been previously published (McCarthy, Jarrett, and Crawley 2001, 902–07). Nonetheless, at this time there are no universally accepted reference values for waist circumference measurements in children. As such, there are no current professional recommendations around obtaining or tracking waist circumference in this younger population (Barlow 2007).

Assessing Body Fat

When it comes to assessing a patient's weight status, clinicians are more concerned with excess weight from adipose or fat mass than with excess weight from lean body mass. Given that BMI does not account for actual fat mass and only serves as a proxy for body fatness, clinicians should use additional measurements when possible to measure body fat. As mentioned, waist circumference is a good indicator for central adiposity, or android obesity. However, if a clinician needed to estimate actual fat mass, additional anthropometrics would need to be obtained.

The gold standard for obtaining a patient's percent body fat is done using a Dual Energy X-Ray Absorptiomtetry (DEXA) scan. This scan is able to distinguish body fat, muscle, and bone mineral, and generates weight and percentage estimates for each of these three compartments. When having the scan done, the patient will need to wear light clothing or an examination gown and will lie supine on the scanner's table, or platform, for ~6 minutes. A report is generated shortly after the scan has completed. Although the use of a DEXA scan is the most preferred method of obtaining body fat percentages, this piece of equipment is extremely expensive and is not portable. As such, it is typically only found in sports medicine clinics and research facilities.

An individual's body fat percentage can also be obtained using hydrostatic, or underwater, weighing. In this procedure, an individual is weighed both on land and while submerged under water, and calculations involving the difference between these two weights estimate his body fat percentage. When making the calculation, the clinician must also take into account residual volume, or the amount of air left in the individual's lungs after maximal expiration, because this will affect the individual's buoyancy and resulting underwater weight. Like the DEXA scan procedure, hydrostatic weighing requires large, heavy equipment and is typically only found in specialized clinics and research facilities.

In clinics without DEXA scans or hydrostatic weighing chambers, clinicians often resort to using bioelectrical impedance analysis (BIA or skinfold measurements) to assess a patient's body fat percentage. BIA is a method by which fat-free mass and total body water can be distinguished from fat mass by passing an electric current through the body (Kyle et al. 2004a, 1226–43). Equipment for BIA is relatively inexpensive and portable; however, strict procedures must be followed, and results should be interpreted with caution given they can be skewed by hydration status and extreme BMI (Kyle et al. 2004b, 1430–53).

Skinfold measurements are also inexpensive and relatively easy to obtain. However, the major assumption when using skinfolds is that the subcutaneous fat being captured by this measurement (or these multiple measurements) is indicative of all body fat, including visceral fat. This may not always be the case. In addition, both within-clinician and between-clinician errors can occur when a patient's skin is either too flaccid or too firm (Lukaski 1987, 537–56), demonstrating the high probability of obtaining incorrect measurements. If skinfolds are taken, they should be done using calibrated calipers across multiple areas of the body. These areas include the triceps, biceps, subscapular region, suprailiac region, midaxillary region (Lohman, Roche, and Martorell 1988). It is important to measure all of these sites because no one region can serve as a proxy for the body's subcutaneous fat layer (Siervogel et al. 1982, 162–71). Although skinfolds are considered appropriate for adults, they are not recommended for assessment of obesity in children (Barlow 2007).

Biochemical Indicators

A clinical diagnosis of overweight or obesity is not typically dependent on a biochemical indicator or laboratory value. However, it is important to note that overweight and obesity are closely correlated with a myriad of chronic diseases, which do have corresponding biochemical indicators. As such, this section will focus on biochemical indicators and laboratory tests, which may help identify patients who would benefit from weight management guidance.

Glucose and Associated Indicators

Overweight and obesity are strong risk factors for prediabetes and type 2 diabetes mellitus (Chan et al. 1994, 961–69; Colditz et al. 1995, 481–86; Dunstan et al. 2002, 829–34), conditions in which blood sugar cannot be properly metabolized. There are a myriad of proposed mechanisms by which the excess adipose tissue disrupts normal glucose metabolism and causes elevated levels of glucose and insulin to remain in the bloodstream. As such, overweight and obese individuals seeking weight management guidance may have abnormal laboratory values associated with glucose and insulin metabolism.

Table 4.2 describes common laboratory tests conducted for those individuals at risk for and who have been diagnosed with prediabetes or type 2 diabetes. Not all clinics will perform all of these tests, these are the ones most commonly ordered in clinical practice. Their associated reference values are also provided.

Table 4.2 Diabetes-related laboratory tests and reference values

Laboratory test	Reference value
Fasting plasma glucose	Normal: <100 mg/dL Prediabetes: 100–125 mg/dL Diabetes: ≥126 mg/dL
2 hour oral glucose tolerance test	Normal: <140 mg/dL Prediabetes: 140–199 mg/dL Diabetes: ≥200 mg/dL
Hemoglobin A1C (glycosylated hemoglobin)	Normal: <5.7% Prediabetes: 5.7%–6.4% Diabetes: ≥6.5%

Source: American Diabetes Association (2015, S8–16).

Research has shown that reductions in weight can substantially improve blood sugar control and, thereby, reduce the risk of developing diabetes (Hamman et al. 2006, 2102–07). As such, individuals with elevated blood glucose levels (e.g., patients with pre-diabetes or diabetes) could reap substantial benefits from a comprehensive weight loss intervention. As part of the intervention, the aforementioned laboratory tests should be routinely monitored for changes.

Note: Certified diabetes educators are specialized clinicians (e.g., physicians, psychologists, dietitians, nurses, pharmacists, etc.) who focus on educating and treating patients with diabetes. Given these clinicians' familiarity with diabetes treatment modalities and medications, including insulin and oral hypoglycemic agents, it is highly recommended they be consulted as part of the weight management intervention for an individual with diabetes.

Cholesterol

Just as glucose values tend to be altered in overweight and obese individuals than normal weight individuals, blood lipids also tend to be altered. As such, blood lipids should be taken in account when performing a nutrition assessment on patients seeking weight management guidance. The American Heart Association recommends that all individuals over 20 years have their lipids, or complete fasting lipoprotein profiles, checked at least every 4 to 6 years (American Heart Association 2015b).

The components of a full lipid profile include: total blood (or serum) cholesterol, high-density lipoprotein (HDL) cholesterol, low-density lipoprotein (LDL) cholesterol, and triglycerides. The total blood cholesterol is a reflection of the patient's overall lipid profile because it is simply the sum of the HDL cholesterol, the LDL cholesterol, and one-fifth of the triglycerides. LDL cholesterol is the main component of the total blood cholesterol that contributes to the build-up of plaque in the arteries. Typically, treatment of hyperlipidemia or hypercholesterolemia will focus on decreasing LDL cholesterol and increasing HDL cholesterol. Having a high HDL value is advantageous because HDL helps remove cholesterol and other harmful substances from the blood stream. Lastly, triglycerides are the free-floating fat in the bloodstream, which can also

Table 4.3 Target values for fasting lipid panels in adults*

	Target values for adults* (mg/dL)	Acceptable levels for children and adolescents
Total cholesterol	<200 (<180 is optimal [American Heart Association 2015b])	<170
LDL cholesterol	<100	<110
HDL cholesterol	≤60	>45
Triglycerides	<150	0–9 years: <75 10–19 years: <90

**Targets and acceptable values may differ depending on a patient's risk factors and/or medication regimen.*

Source: National Cholesterol Education Program (NCEP) Expert Panel on Detection, Evaluation, and Treatment of High Blood Cholesterol in Adults (Adult Treatment Panel III) (2002, 3143–421) and children/adolescents (U.S. Department of Health and Human Services 2012).

contribute to plaque build-up. Target ranges for all components of the complete fasting lipid profile can be found in Table 4.3.

Additional Biochemical Indicators

As noted in Table 4.4, additional laboratory tests may be conducted on patients suspected of having medical conditions associated with overweight and obesity. Similarly, if a patient has a family history of medical conditions that contribute to weight problems, a clinician may elect to run additional tests.

Because the thyroid gland regulates metabolism and energy expenditure, many clinicians will also evaluate a patient's thyroid stimulating hormone (TSH) and free thyroxine (T4) levels. High levels of TSH and low levels of T4 may indicate hypothyroidism, a condition that can contribute to weight gain. Patients with this underlying condition should be evaluated for medication intervention as well as lifestyle and weight management.

Uric acid is another laboratory test that may be conducted on those patients at high risk for and who have previously been diagnosed with gout. Gout, a complex form of arthritis that is more common in individuals who are overweight or obese, occurs when there is a build-up of urate crystals in body joints. These crystals typically form when uric acid levels in the bloodstream are abnormally high. As such, clinicians can order regular uric acid (blood or urine) tests to monitor a patient's status and risk for having a gout attack.

Table 4.4 Reference values for additional obesity-related biochemical indicators

	Reference values
TSH (U.S. National Library of Medicine, National Institutes of Health 2014b)	0.4–4.0 milli-international units per liter (mIU/L)
Free thyroxine (U.S. National Library of Medicine, National Institutes of Health 2014a)	4.5–11.2 micrograms per deciliter (mg/dL)
Uric acid (blood) (U.S. National Library of Medicine, National Institutes of Health 2013b)	3.5–7.2 mg/dL
Uric acid (urine) (U.S. National Library of Medicine, National Institutes of Health 2013c)	250–750 mg/24 hour
CRP (U.S. National Library of Medicine, National Institutes of Health 2013a)	Low risk: <1.0 mg/L Average risk: 1.0–3.0 mg/L High risk: >3.0 mg/L

C-reactive protein, or CRP, is an acute phase response protein that becomes elevated during inflammation. Elevated levels of CRP are associated with many of the chronic diseases seen in overweight and obese individuals, such as type 2 diabetes, cardiovascular disease, and hypertension. As such, clinicians may elect to monitor CRP levels in these individuals, although this is not routinely recommended until the patient is considered high risk.

Physical Signs and Symptoms

In a typical nutrition assessment, clinical signs and symptoms are used to identify signs of malnutrition and nutritional deficiency among patients seeking nutritional guidance. However, given that most patients seeking weight management guidance already consume sufficient nutrients and calories, the attending clinician may rely more heavily on data gathered as part of the anthropometric, biochemical, and dietary intake assessments and less on the clinical or physical assessment. Nonetheless, there are some clinical signs and symptoms that, when present, should be documented as support for weight management intervention.

Blood Pressure

Blood pressure is a nutrition-focused physical finding that is useful to monitor and apply during the nutrition assessment process. The association between blood pressure and weight status has been documented in both adults and children (Muntner et al. 2004, 2107–13), thus making blood pressure a relevant laboratory value to include as part of the nutritional assessment of patients who desire weight management guidance. Just as weight loss can reduce plasma glucose levels and the risk of diabetes, it can also help improve blood pressure in individuals with prehypertension and hypertension (National Heart Lung and Blood Institute 1998; Whelton et al. 1998, 839–46).

Table 4.5 displays the reference values for normal blood pressure, prehypertension, and the various stages of hypertension. These values should be taken into consideration when assessing a patient for a weight management program, and blood pressure should be monitored as part of a comprehensive program.

Body Shape

As mentioned in the earlier section on anthropometrics, patients who appear to carry their excess weight in the body's abdominal region (i.e., the android shape) are more at-risk for chronic health problems than those who carry excess weight in the body's extremities (i.e., the gynoid shape). In patients who are overweight and obese, these two shapes may be identified through clinical observation. However, clinicians should be

Table 4.5 American Heart Association's blood pressure categories

	Systolic reading		Diastolic reading
Normal	<120 mm Hg	*and*	<80 mm Hg
Prehypertension	120 139 mm Hg	*or*	80–89 mm Hg
Hypertension: Stage I	140–159 mm Hg	*or*	90–99 mm Hg
Hypertension: Stage II	≥160 mm Hg	*or*	≥100 mm Hg
Hypertensive Crisis (*emergency care warranted*)	>180 mm Hg	*or*	>110 mm Hg

Source: American Heart Association (2015a).

aware that bulky and loose clothing can skew this observation, thus making measurements, such as waist circumference, important in diagnosing android versus gynoid obesity.

Acanthosis Nigricans

Another clinical manifestation associated with excess weight is acanthosis nigricans. This condition is characterized by a darkening of the patient's skin in areas where the skin naturally folds, such as around the neck and under the arms. Acanthosis nigricans is commonly seen in patients with impaired glucose tolerance and insulin resistance, and those patients are also likely to be overweight or obese. As such, weight loss is typically prescribed as part of a comprehensive medical treatment plan to ameliorate this condition.

Additional Physical Findings

Other physical findings that should be noted as part of the nutrition assessment include:

- Amputations or other limitations to physical functionality
- Communication impairments (e.g., hearing, speech)
- Disposition and body language
- Heart rate
- Missing teeth or poor dentition

If any of the aforementioned clinical characteristics are found to be abnormal, the success of a weight management program could be compromised. As such, the clinician should consider making additional medical referrals prior to implementing a weight management program.

Patient Interview

Although data gathered as part of the anthropometric, biochemical and physical assessments are important to the overall nutrition assessment, critical information is also gathered during the patient interview. It is during this process of the assessment that the patient's usual dietary intake and related behaviors are revealed. Additional information on the patient's medical, social, and family history can also be garnered as part of this process. All of this information must be taken into consideration when tailoring a comprehensive weight management program.

Dietary Intake

A critical part of the nutrition assessment involves the assessment of the patient's normal dietary intake. When possible, a dietary intake assessment should be performed by a Registered Dietitian Nutritionist (RDN) (Academy of Nutrition and Dietetics 2014), as RDNs are specifically trained to accurately measure energy and nutrient intake using validated dietary assessment methods. The assessment can be made using a number of methods, including a single or multiple 24 hour dietary recalls, a food record, or a food frequency questionnaire (FFQ). Although there are additional methods of collecting dietary intake data (e.g., capturing photos of foods consumed, direct observation), only the three aforementioned techniques will be described in brief detail.

Twenty-Four Hour Dietary Recalls

Twenty-four hour dietary recalls are commonly used when a clinician seeks to understand a patient's most recent dietary intake. A 24 hour recall captures what and how much a patient has eaten over the previous 24 hour time period. In some cases, however, a clinician may prefer to capture this information by asking a patient what he consumed from 12:00 a.m. to 11:59 p.m. on the previous day (as opposed to simply asking about dietary intake over the preceding 24 hours). This latter technique may be easier for the patient to recall and is commonly used when gathering 24 hour dietary recall information for large-scale nutrition surveys (U.S. Department of Health and Human Services, Centers for Disease Control and Prevention 2013).

When collecting a 24 hour dietary recall for research purposes, the process should be guided by an automated computer software program. However, given this software is expensive and rarely available in most clinical practices, clinicians will most likely gather this recall information using verbal guidance.

When collecting the recall, the clinician should ask probing questions that elicit a thorough response from the patient. Thorough responses should include the specific type and amount of food consumed as well as any beverages consumed along with the food. The clinician should be careful to avoid asking leading questions that might provoke a specific response from the patient (i.e., "Are you sure you didn't eat any fruits or vegetables yesterday?"). The clinician should also avoid the use of judgmental terms when collecting information on the patient's intake, as this could inhibit a truthful and accurate response.

Most clinicians find it helpful to have food models available when collecting the 24 hour recall. These food models assist the patient in more accurately recalling the amounts of foods and beverages consumed. These models also can also serve as a good reference size when discussing portion control during the weight management intervention.

In addition to collecting information about what and how much food and beverage were consumed, the clinician should also ask the patient where he consumed his foods. This information will provide insight into the environments where he normally eats and can provide a rationale for the foods being consumed.

There are several limitations to using a 24 hour dietary recall when assessing a patient's dietary intake. First, the 24 hour timeframe captured in this recall may not accurately reflect a patient's usual intake. For this reason, clinicians may want to capture multiple 24 hour recalls then average the intake over those multiple recalls to deduce the patient's usual intake.

In addition, some patients may have difficulty with accurately recalling what they consumed. This is especially true for patients with memory impairment or psychological disorders. Young patients may also have difficulty with accurately recalling what and how much they consumed. If there are other individuals who may be able to supplement the patient's recall (i.e., a parent or caregiver), then those individuals should be asked to participate in the recall collection. However, patients must first consent to having these individuals present during the interview.

Food Records

Another technique for gathering dietary assessment data is the use of a food record. A food record is simply a log of the foods and beverages a patient consumed over a specified period of time. Whether a record is kept for 3 days or for 3 months, a food record may contain more accurate information than the 24 hour dietary recall and may provide a more accurate depiction of usual dietary intake.

Typically, a patient will receive a blank food record via mail or e-mail prior to his visit with the clinician. The food record should include detailed instructions on how to keep the record, or an instructional phone call should be conducted with the patient. Giving the patient detailed instructions will ensure accurate and thorough documentation and will allow for a full analysis to be conducted once the food record is returned to the clinician.

Each page of a food record should represent its own day. For example, Monday's and Tuesday's intakes should be recorded on separate records. Each record should include at least the following elements: day, time and meal, location, food or beverage consumed, and amount consumed. Gathering information on these elements is important as it allows the clinician to easily identify trends in intake (e.g., eating breakfast in the car, having large gaps in time between meals) and it allows the clinician to analyze intake for nutrients and food groups.

A major limitation to the food record is the burden of collecting this information. Patients may find it difficult to write down everything they eat and drink for multiple days at a time. In addition, patients can still forget to document all the foods and beverages they eat, particularly if they are not consumed at a time when the patient can document their intake (e.g., while riding in a car, while sitting in a meeting). All of these conditions may lead to inaccurate reporting and analysis and should be considered when deciding how to assess a patient's diet.

Food Frequency Questionnaires

FFQs are another technique used to assess a patient's dietary intake. Whereas the 24 hour recall and food record ask a patient to document what he consumes, FFQs simply ask a series of questions that the patient answers using a multiple choice option. FFQs also tend to be focused on specific nutrients or food groups (e.g., sodium, fruits, and vegetables) rather than the full dietary intake; thus they may not fully describe a patient's entire dietary intake.

The benefit of using an FFQ is that it captures a patient's usual intake without asking him or her to specifically recall what he or she ate on a certain day or days. For example, an FFQ may ask "How frequently do you eat bananas?" and the answer options may range from two to three times per day to less than once per year. This dietary assessment method allows a patient to take into consideration seasonal variation in food intake.

FFQs can range in length from one to several pages, making some of the longer versions more time-intensive to complete. Nonetheless, if they are focused on specific nutrients or food groups, this will shorten the length of the questionnaire and allow the patient to complete it in a short time period. These shorter questionnaires may be advantageous for clinicians who ask their patients to complete the assessment upon arriving for an appointment.

If clinicians wish to use an FFQ in their practice, they should only use previously validated and reliable FFQs that have been tested on their specific patient population. For example, an FFQ that has been validated in adults should not be used for children, and vice versa. In addition, it is most advantageous to use an FFQ in conjunction with a 24 hour dietary recall (or recalls) or a detailed food record in order to assess a patient's usual dietary intake. This is especially true for patients requesting weight management guidance as most FFQs will not accurately access average caloric intake when used alone.

Historical Data

Because of the myriad comorbidities associated with overweight and obesity, the medical history of patients seeking weight management guidance should be fully explored. It is important to note that there are multiple medical conditions in which weight management or weight loss may be contraindicated (e.g., patient with eating disorders, pregnant women, patients undergoing treatment for cancer). As such, clinicians should ensure the weight management program is appropriate.

This historical data, along with other pertinent information, can be acquired during the patient interview. Box 4.1 outlines some questions that should be posed during the interview process.

Box 4.1 Example questions to ask during the patient interview portion of the nutrition assessment

Medical history

- What medical conditions have you been diagnosed with or treated for in the past?
- What medical conditions are you currently being treated for? (Obtain contact information for the attending clinician if needed)
- What medications are you currently taking?
- What allergies, including food allergies, do you have?

Weight history:

- What is the least you have ever weighed in your adult life? What is the most?
- How long have you been at your current weight?
- What patterns in weight fluctuation have you noticed over the years?
- What affects your weight? Does stress tend to make you gain or lose weight?

Social history

- Tell me about your current living situation. Who resides with you?
- Tell me about your current employment or school situation.
- Tell me about your income status. Do you have enough money to buy food?
- How often do you smoke cigarettes? How many do you smoke each day or week?
- How often do you consume alcohol? How much do you consume on each occasion? (Include as part of the dietary assessment as well)

(*Continued*)

(*Continued*)

Family history

- What is your family's history of overweight or obesity?
- What is your family's history of heart disease? Diabetes? Cancer?
- What is your family's history of psychiatric illness (e.g., depression, anxiety)?

Psychological history

- Have you ever been seen by a psychiatrist, counselor, or therapist?
- Have you ever taken medication for anxiety, stress, depression, or another mental health condition?
- Has anyone, including you, ever suspected you had an eating disorder?
- How would you describe your relationship with food?

Beliefs and Attitudes

As discussed in Chapter 3, an individual's food-related beliefs and attitudes can significantly impact his food choices. During the patient's interview, clinicians should inquire about patient's beliefs around food and nutrition and how these beliefs are formed. In some cases, religious principles will shape an individual's food beliefs and preferences (e.g., Muslims may fast during Ramadan; Catholics may avoid red meat on Fridays). In other cases, environmental or humanitarian beliefs may shape an individual's preferences (e.g., environmental activists may prefer to only consume local, sustainably grown foods).

Food beliefs and preferences may also be impacted by a patient's previous experiences. For example, an individual who has been a chronic or yo-yo dieter may be less motivated to follow a meal plan if he has failed at dieting in the past. A patient who has tried a multitude of fad diets may also be less motivated to follow a healthy diet plan and may be more inclined to follow the newest fad. These previous experiences can affect motivation and adherence; thus it is important for the clinician to understand them prior to enrolling the patient in a weight management program.

Summary

The nutrition assessment process is an important first step when providing weight management guidance. A full assessment takes into account a patient's anthropometric measurements, biochemical factors, and physical signs as well as information gathered during an interview. Together, these elements will reveal the patient's current nutritional status and provide rationale for or against weight management interventions.

References

Academy of Nutrition and Dietetics. 2014. "Adult Weight Management: Executive Summary of Recommendations." www.andeal.org/topic.cfm?menu=5276&cat=4690 (accessed July 2, 2015).

American Diabetes Association. 2015. "(2) Classification and Diagnosis of Diabetes." *Diabetes Care* 38, Suppl. 1, pp. S8–16. doi:10.2337/dc15-S005

American Heart Association. 2015a. "Understanding Blood Pressure Readings." www.heart.org/HEARTORG/Conditions/HighBloodPressure/AboutHighBloodPressure/Understanding-Blood-Pressure-Readings_UCM_301764_Article.jsp (accessed May 30, 2015).

American Heart Association. 2015b. "What Your Cholesterol Levels Mean." www.heart.org/HEARTORG/Conditions/Cholesterol/AboutCholesterol/What-Your-Cholesterol-Levels-Mean_UCM_305562_Article.jsp (accessed May 30, 2015).

Barlow, S.E. 2007. "Expert Committee and Treatment of Child and Adolescent Overweight and Obesity: Expert Committee Recommendations regarding the Prevention." *Assessment, Report Pediatrics* 120.

Beker, L. 2006. "Principles of Growth Assessment." *Pediatrics in Review/American Academy of Pediatrics* 27, no. 5, pp. 196–98. doi:10.1542/pir.27-5-196

Bjorntorp, P. 1987. "Classification of Obese Patients and Complications Related to the Distribution of Surplus Fat." *American Journal of Clinical Nutrition (USA)* 45, pp. 1120–25.

Chan, J.M., E.B. Rimm, G.A. Colditz, M.J. Stampfer, and W.C. Willett. 1994. "Obesity, Fat Distribution, and Weight Gain as Risk Factors for Clinical Diabetes in Men." *Diabetes Care* 17, no. 9, pp. 961–69. doi:10.2337/diacare.17.9.961

Chumlea, W.C., A.F. Roche, and M.L. Steinbaugh. 1985. "Estimating Stature from Knee Height for Persons 60 to 90 Years of Age," *Journal of the American Geriatrics Society* 33, no. 2, pp. 116–20. doi:10.1111/j.1532-5415.1985.tb02276.x

Chumlea, W.M.C., S.S. Guo, and M.L. Steinbaugh. 1994. "Prediction of Stature from Knee Height for Black and White Adults and Children with Application to Mobility-Impaired or Handicapped Persons." *Journal of the American Dietetic Association* 94, no. 12, pp. 1385–91. doi:10.1016/0002-8223(94)92540-2

Colditz, G.A., W.C. Willett, A. Rotnitzky, and J.E. Manson. 1995. "Weight Gain as a Risk Factor for Clinical Diabetes Mellitus in Women." *Annals of Internal Medicine* 122, no. 7, pp. 481–86. doi:10.7326/0003-4819-122-7-199504010-00001

Czernichow, S., A.-P. Kengne, E. Stamatakis, M. Hamer, and G.D. Batty. 2011. "Body Mass Index, Waist Circumference and Waist–Hip Ratio: Which Is the Better Discriminator of Cardiovascular Disease Mortality Risk? Evidence from an Individual-Participant Meta-Analysis of 82 864 Participants from Nine Cohort Studies." *Obesity Reviews* 12, no. 9, pp. 680–87. doi:10.1111/j.1467-789x.2011.00879.x

de Koning, L., A.T. Merchant, J. Pogue, and S.S. Anand. 2007. "Waist Circumference and Waist-to-Hip Ratio as Predictors of Cardiovascular Events: Meta-Regression Analysis of Prospective Studies." *European Heart Journal* 28, no. 7, pp. 850–56. doi:10.1093/eurheartj/ehm026

de Onis, M. 2006. WHO Child Growth Standards: Length/Height-for-Age, Weight-for-Age, Weight-for-Length, Weight-for-Height and Body Mass Index-for-Age, Geneva, World Health Organization.

Dunstan, D.W., P.Z. Zimmet, T.A. Welborn, M.P. De Courten, A.J. Cameron, R.A. Sicree, T. Dwyer, S. Colagiuri, D. Jolley, M. Knuiman, R. Atkins, and J.E. Shaw. 2002. "The Rising Prevalence of Diabetes and Impaired Glucose Tolerance: The Australian Diabetes, Obesity and Lifestyle Study." *Diabetes Care* 25, no. 5, pp. 829–34. doi:10.2337/diacare.25.5.829

Flegal, K.M., J.A. Shepherd, A.C. Looker, B.I. Graubard, L.G. Borrud, C.L. Ogden, T.B. Harris, J.E. Everhart, and N. Schenker. 2009. "Comparisons of Percentage Body Fat, Body Mass Index, Waist Circumference, and Waist-Stature Ratio in Adults." *The American Journal of Clinical Nutrition* 89, no. 2, pp. 500–08. doi:10.3945/ajcn.2008.26847

Freedman, D.S., M. Horlick, and G.S. Berenson. 2013. "A Comparison of the Slaughter Skinfold-Thickness Equations and BMI in Predicting Body Fatness and Cardiovascular Disease Risk Factor Levels in Children." *The American Journal of Clinical Nutrition* 98, no. 6, pp. 1417–24. doi:10.3945/ajcn.113.065961

Garrow, J.S., and J. Webster. 1985. "Quetelet's Index (W/H2) as a Measure of Fatness." *International Journal of Obesity* 9, no. 2, pp. 147–53.

Hamman, R.F., R.R. Wing, S.L. Edelstein, J.M. Lachin, G.A. Bray, L. Delahanty, M. Hoskin, A.M. Kriska, E.J. Mayer-Davis, X. Pi-Sunyer, J. Regensteiner, B. Venditti, J. Wylie-Rosett, and for the Diabetes Prevention Program Research Group. 2006. "Effect of Weight Loss with Lifestyle Intervention on Risk of Diabetes." *Diabetes Care* 29, no. 9, pp. 2102–7. doi:10.2337/dc06-0560

Jarzem, P.F., and R.B. Gledhill. 1993. "Predicting Height from Arm Measurements." *Journal of Pediatric Orthopaedics* 13, no. 6, pp. 761–65. doi:10.1097/01241398-199311000-00014

Kyle, U.G., I. Bosaeus, A.D. De Lorenzo, P. Deurenberg, M. Elia, J.M. Gómez, B.L. Heitmann, L. Kent-Smith, J.-C. Melchior, M. Pirlich, H. Scharfetter, A.M.W.J. Schols, and C. Pichard. 2004a. "Bioelectrical Impedance Analysis—Part I: Review of Principles and Methods." *Clinical Nutrition* 23, no. 5, pp. 1226–43. doi:10.1016/j.clnu.2004.06.004

Kyle, U.G., I. Bosaeus, A.D. De Lorenzo, P. Deurenberg, M. Elia, J.M. Gómez, B.L. Heitmann, L. Kent-Smith, J.-C. Melchior, M. Pirlich, H. Scharfetter, A.M.W.J. Schols, and C. Pichard. 2004b. "Bioelectrical Impedance Analysis—Part II: Utilization in Clinical Practice." *Clinical Nutrition* 23, no. 6, pp. 1430–53. doi:10.1016/j.clnu.2004.09.012

Lee, S., F. Bacha, N. Gungor, and S.A. Arslanian. 2006. "Waist Circumference Is an Independent Predictor of Insulin Resistance in Black and White Youths." *The Journal of Pediatrics* 148, no. 2, pp. 188–94. doi:10.1016/j.jpeds.2005.10.001

Lohman, T.G., A.F. Roche, and R. Martorell. 1988. *Anthropometric Standardization Reference Manual.* Champaign, IL: Human Kinetics Books.

Lukaski, H.C. 1987. "Methods for the Assessment of Human Body Composition: Traditional and New." *The American Journal of Clinical Nutrition* 46, no. 4, pp. 537–56.

Maffeis, C., A. Pietrobelli, A. Grezzani, S. Provera, and L. Tatò. 2001. "Waist Circumference and Cardiovascular Risk Factors in Prepubertal Children." *Obesity Research* 9, no. 3, pp. 179–87. doi:10.1038/oby.2001.19

McCarthy, H.D., K.V. Jarrett, and H.F. Crawley. 2001. "Original Communications-the Development of Waist Circumference Percentiles in British Children Aged 5.0-16.9 y." *European Journal of Clinical Nutrition* 55, no. 10, pp. 902–7. doi:10.1038/sj.ejcn.1601240

Mechanick, J.I., A. Youdim, D.B. Jones, W.T. Garvey, D.L. Hurley, M.M. McMahon, L.J. Heinberg, R. Kushner, T.D. Adams, S. Shikora, J.B. Dixon, and S. Brethauer. 2013. "Clinical Practice Guidelines for the Perioperative Nutritional, Metabolic, and Nonsurgical Support of the Bariatric Surgery patient—2013 Update: Cosponsored by American Association of Clinical Endocrinologists, the Obesity Society, and American Society for Metabolic & Bariatric Surgery." *Obesity* 21, no. S1, pp. S1–27.

Muntner, P., J. He, J.A. Cutler, R.P. Wildman, and P.K. Whelton. 2004. "Trends in Blood Pressure among Children and Adolescents." *Jama* 291, no. 17, pp. 2107–13. doi:10.1001/jama.291.17.2107

National Cholesterol Education Program (NCEP) Expert Panel on Detection, Evaluation, and Treatment of High Blood Cholesterol in Adults (Adult Treatment Panel III). 2002. "Third Report of the National Cholesterol Education Program (NCEP) Expert Panel on Detection, Evaluation, and Treatment of High Blood Cholesterol in Adults (Adult Treatment Panel III) Final Report." *Circulation* 106, no. 25, pp. 3143–421.

National Heart Lung and Blood Institute. 1998. Clinical Guidelines on the Identification, Evaluation, and Treatment of Overweight and Obesity in Adults, NIH Publication no. 98-4083, National Institutes of Health.

Roche, A.F., and G.H. Davila. 1974. "Differences Between Recumbent Length and Stature within Individuals." *Growth* 38, no. 3, pp. 313–20.

Savva, S.C., M. Tornaritis, M.E. Savva, Y. Kourides, A. Panagi, N. Silikiotou, C. Georgiou, and A. Kafatos. 2000. "Waist Circumference and Waist-to-Height Ratio Are Better Predictors of Cardiovascular Disease Risk Factors in Children than Body Mass Index." *International Journal of Obesity and Related Metabolic Disorders: Journal of the International Association for the Study of Obesity* 24, no. 11, pp. 1453–58. doi:10.1038/sj.ijo.0801401

Siervogel, R.M., A.F. Roche, J.H. Himes, W.C. Chumlea, and R. McCammon. 1982. "Subcutaneous Fat Distribution in Males and Females from 1 to 39 Years of Age." *The American Journal of Clinical Nutrition* 36, no. 1, pp. 162–71.

Stallings, V.A., and B.S. Zemel. 1996. "Nutrition Assessment of the Disabled Child." In *Clinics in Developmental Medicine: Feeding the Disabled Child*, eds. P.B. Sullivan and R. Rosenbloom, 62. London: Mackeith Press.

Steele, M.F., and T.C. Chenier. 1990. "Arm-Span, Height, and Age in Black and White Women." *Annals of Human Biology* 17, no. 6, pp. 533–41. doi:10.1080/03014469000001312

U.S. Department of Health and Human Services. 2012. "Integrated Guidelines for Cardiovascular Health and Risk Reduction in Children and Adolescents." www.nhlbi.nih.gov/health-pro/guidelines/current/cardiovascular-health-pediatric-guidelines

U.S. Department of Health and Human Services, Centers for Disease Control and Prevention. 2013. "National Health and Nutrition Examination Survey (NHANES): Anthropometry Procedures Manual." www.cdc.gov/nchs/data/nhanes/nhanes_13_14/2013_Anthropometry.pdf (accessed May 25, 2015).

U.S. Department of Health and Human Services, Centers for Disease Control and Prevention, National Center for Health Statistics. 2010a. "Growth Charts - Homepage." www.cdc.gov/growthcharts/index.htm (accessed June 2, 2015).

U.S. Department of Health and Human Services, Centers for Disease Control and Prevention, National Center for Health Statistics. 2010b. "Growth Charts - WHO Growth Standards Are Recommended for Use in the US for Infants and Children 0 to 2 Years of Age." www.cdc.gov/growthcharts/who_charts.htm#The%20WHO%20Growth%20Charts (accessed June 2, 2015).

U.S. National Library of Medicine, National Institutes of Health. 2013a. "C-Reactive Protein: Medline Plus Medical Encyclopedia." www.nlm.nih.gov/medlineplus/ency/article/003356.htm (accessed May 30, 2015).

U.S. National Library of Medicine, National Institutes of Health. 2013b. "Uric Acid-Blood: Medline Plus Medical Encyclopedia." www.nlm.nih.gov/medlineplus/ency/article/003476.htm (accessed May 30, 2015).

U.S. National Library of Medicine, National Institutes of Health. 2013c. "Uric Acid-Urine: Medline Plus Medical Encyclopedia." www.nlm.nih.gov/medlineplus/ency/article/003616.htm (accessed May 30, 2015).

U.S. National Library of Medicine, National Institutes of Health. 2014a. "T4 Test: Medline Plus Medical Encyclopedia." www.nlm.nih.gov/medlineplus/ency/article/003517.htm (accessed May 30, 2015).

U.S. National Library of Medicine, National Institutes of Health. 2014b. "TSH Test: Medline Plus Medical Encyclopedia." www.nlm.nih.gov/medlineplus/ency/article/003684.htm (accessed May 30, 2015).

Whelton, P.K., L.J. Appel, M.A. Espeland, W.B. Applegate, W.H. Ettinger Jr, J.B. Kostis, S. Kumanyika, C.R. Lacy, K.C. Johnson, S. Folmar, J.A. Cutler, and for the TONE Collaborative Research Group. 1998. "Sodium Reduction and Weight Loss in the Treatment of Hypertension in Older Persons: A Randomized Controlled Trial of Nonpharmacologic Interventions in the Elderly (TONE)." *Jama* 279, no. 11, pp. 839–46. doi:10.1001/jama.279.11.839

Wohlfahrt-Veje, C., J. Tinggaard, K. Winther, A. Mouritsen, C.P. Hagen, M.G. Mieritz, K.T. de Renzy-Martin, M. Boas, J.H. Petersen, and K.M. Main. 2014. "Body Fat Throughout Childhood in 2647 Healthy Danish Children: Agreement of BMI, Waist Circumference, Skinfolds with Dual X-Ray Absorptiometry." *European Journal of Clinical Nutrition* 68, no. 6, pp. 664–70. doi:10.1038/ejcn.2013.282

World Health Organization (WHO). 1995. Physical Status: The Use of and Interpretation of Anthropometry, Report of a WHO Expert Committee., Technical Report Series No. 854.

WHO. 2008. Waist Circumference and Waist-Hip Ratio. Report of a WHO Expert Consultation, Geneva, World Health Organization, December 8–11.

CHAPTER 5

Weight Loss Intervention: Program Characteristics and Components

A comprehensive weight management program will exhibit a myriad of characteristics and include many components that have the potential to impact a patient's success. In this chapter, program characteristics and components will be explored using a who/what/when/where approach.

The "Who" Component: Who Should Be Involved?

The first major component of a weight management program is the people involved in the program. Although the patient and clinicians are the primary individuals involved, family and friends who provide social support should also be included as long as the patient consents to their involvement.

Patient

The patient should always be at the center of the weight management program, and his needs and behaviors should steer the direction of his individualized program. As outlined in Chapter 4, a full assessment of a patient's needs should be performed prior to a patient entering a weight management program, and the findings from this assessment should establish a foundation on which the weight management program is built.

Keeping the patient at the center of the program seems intuitive given that the patient is the one enrolled in the program. However, at times this can be difficult. This is especially true when a clinician is trying to meet certain standards or when the clinician's resources are limited. For example, many clinicians have quotas for the number of patients they need to see each day. Although it is important to meet this quota, it is also important to not allow this time crunch to interfere with the quality of time spent with a patient. To avoid feeling rushed and to keep the patient at the center of the visit, the clinician can alert the patient to his time limitations prior to the visit so that the time can be well-spent on topics pertinent to the patient's success.

Registered Dietitian Nutritionist

Because nutrition and dietary intake are at the core of any weight management program, a Registered Dietitian Nutrition (RDN) should be the primary treating clinician and should spearhead the intervention. RDNs are extensively trained in creating energy-restricted meal plans and have expertise in modifying these plans as needed. They also have training in physical and dietary assessment as well as in behavior modification. Because their skills are essential to a success weight management program, the RDN is the most appropriate clinician to oversee the weight management intervention.

Multidisciplinary Team

Although the RDN should spearhead the intervention, other members of the patient's medical team should also be involved in the weight management program. The medical team will typically include the primary care physician (PCP) as well as other physicians, nurse practitioners, or physician assistants who oversee the patient's medical care. Although these individuals do not need to be involved with every visit, they should be kept abreast of the patient's progress and be encouraged to provide input and feedback when necessary. Often times, the primary contact on the patient's medical team will participate in the weight management program by writing orders for laboratory tests or prescription medications.

For patients with chronic illnesses, additional specialists may need to be included on the medical team. In patients with diabetes, the patient's endocrinologist would be an essential member of the team, as he would need to monitor the patient's glucose levels as the patient loses weight and becomes more physically active. In patients with cardiovascular disease (CVD), the patient's cardiologist would need to be involved in the weight management program. Because blood pressure responds fairly rapidly to weight loss, the cardiologist may need to adjust the patient's blood pressure medications (e.g., angiotensin-converting-enzyme (ACE) inhibitors, diuretics, β blockers) in response to changes in body weight. Other specialists who may need to be involved are listed in Box 5.1.

Box 5.1 *Examples of medical providers who could be involved in the weight management program (list is not exhaustive)*

Primary providers:

PCP or other attending physician
Pediatrician (for children)
Nurse or general practitioner
Physician assistant

Specialty providers:

Bariatric surgeon (for patients considering or s/p weight loss surgery)
Cardiologist (for patients with CVD)
Gastroenterologist (for patients with gastrointestinal disorders)
Gerontologist (for older patients)
Endocrinologist or Certified Diabetes Educators (for patients with diabetes or other endocrine disorders)
OBGYN (for any female patient who may be trying to get pregnant)
Psychologist or Psychiatrist (for patient undergoing psychiatric treatment)
Rheumatologists (for patients with arthritis or related conditions)

Ancillary providers:

Case and/or social worker
Diabetes educator
Exercise physiologist
Physical therapist
Occupational therapist

Supporters

When appropriate, family and friends who provide social support to the patient can be involved in the weight management program (McLean et al. 2003, 987–1005). Their involvement may depend on their availability and the patient's desire to have them involved, but to the extent possible and beneficial, they may be included as part of the treatment program. Research has shown that when friends and family are included in weight loss program, patients are likely to lose more weight and be more successful at keeping the weight off than when participating in interventions alone (Wing and Jeffery 1999, 132). This is especially true among females, who have been shown to have greater weight loss when they have the support of family and friends (Kiernan et al. 2012, 756–64), and among young children ages 6 to 12 years (Academy of Nutrition and Dietetics 2007, 11).

Social support can also come in the form of group therapy or group interventions. Including a support group as part of the weight loss programs has been found particularly helpful among patients who have undergone weight loss surgery. As such, postsurgical support groups are now an integral part of weight loss surgical treatment.

The "What" Component: What Should Be Included?

Just as energy balance is largely influenced by energy intake (diet) and expenditure (physical activity), diet and physical activity are two central components of a weight management program (Academy of Nutrition and Dietetics 2014). In addition, a behavior modification component should also be included in order to detect any underlying psycho-social contributors to dietary and activity-related behaviors.

Dietary Component

The dietary component of any weight management program should focus on creating a caloric deficit. As mentioned, a caloric deficit of 500 to 750 kcal/day should be one of the dietary goals as it is sufficient to induce weight loss. This caloric deficit can be met using a variety of approaches, several of which are discussed in detail in Chapter 7.

The dietary component of the weight management program should be directed by an RDN who creates meal plans and instructs the patient on how to follow an energy-restricted diet. The RDN may also teach the patient (and possibly his family) how to reduce caloric intake by using various food preparation methods or by controlling portion sizes. Additional strategies used by the RDN are explored in later chapters in this textbook.

Physical Activity Component

Because physical activity is the main modifiable factor in energy expenditure, it is also a primary component of the weight management program. Guidance pertaining to daily activity and exercise should be individualized and based on the patient's current activity level and physical abilities. Because overweight and obese individuals are at an increased risk for chronic disease, medical clearance should be obtained prior to prescribing and initiating a physical activity regimen. In addition, credentialed healthcare clinicians who specialize in exercise and physical activity (e.g., exercise physiologists, physical therapists, and sports medicine physicians) should be included as part of the multidisciplinary team and consulted as needed. Additional information on physical activity can be found in Chapter 12.

Behavioral Modification

The third integral component of a weight management program is the behavioral modification component. Dietary intake and physical activity are both learned behaviors that can be influenced by a range of factors, many of which were outlined in Chapter 3.

The behavioral modification component of a weight management program is the component that focuses on sustainable behavior changes. These changes may be directly related to diet and physical activity, or they can also be related to the factors that influence diet and physical activity such as controlling stressful situations. Strategies to conduct this component are discussed in Chapter 9.

The "When" Component: When Should the Program Take Place?

Early Intervention

Ideally, the weight management program should be initiated when a patient is first detected as being overweight. This is known as early intervention. The Academy of Nutrition and Dietetics currently recommends that clinicians screen their adult patients for their weight status (i.e., obtain height, weight, and waist circumference) at least annually (Academy of Nutrition and Dietetics 2014). Similarly, it is recommended that clinicians annually screen pediatric patients (ages 2 years and older) for BMI and weight status (Barlow 2007; Krebs, Jacobson, and American Academy of Pediatrics Committee on Nutrition 2003, 424–30; U.S. Department of Health and Human Services, Centers for Disease Control and Prevention 2015). If a patient is found to be overweight during a screening visit, then the clinician should immediately refer the patient to a weight management program for early intervention and treatment.

The problem, however, is that not all patients are seen by a healthcare clinician every year. In 2012, roughly 18 percent of adults had not seen a doctor or other healthcare professional in over a year (Blackwell, Lucas, and Clarke 2014, 1–161). If patients are not being seen and screened on a regular basis, then early intervention may not be possible.

In addition, not all clinicians may find it appropriate or within their abilities to screen patients for weight status. This may be a result of the clinician's specialty (e.g., ophthalmologists may not feel comfortable screening for weight because weight-related disorders are outside their scope of practice) or a result of the environment (e.g., emergency room clinicians may not have sufficient time to address a chronic illness such as obesity).

Although early intervention is most desirable, more than 34 percent of adults and nearly 17 percent of children are already obese (Ogden et al. 2014, 806–14), indicating that early intervention has not occurred (or may have not been sufficient) and warranting a comprehensive treatment program to reduce body weight.

Frequency and Duration

In the early phases of an adult weight management program, patients will be focusing on losing weight. As such, the patient should have a minimum of 14 visits with and RDN during at least the first 6 months of the program (Academy of Nutrition and Dietetics 2014). This will ensure the patient is receiving the appropriate guidance and necessary support to facilitate a healthy rate of weight loss. It will also allow the RDN to adequately supervise the process and readily detect and address any problems that arise.

Once the patient has moved onto the weight maintenance phase, visits with the RDN can be less frequent. In this phase, adult patients should continue to meet with the RDN for 12 months, but these visits only need to occur on a monthly basis.

Weight management programs for pediatric patients should last for a minimum of 3 months or until the weight management goals are met (American Dietetic Association 2007). The program's duration may increase for obese children and for those children who do not progress quickly. A greater frequency of visits is also associated with more success in a weight management program; so just as with adult patients, pediatric patients should schedule regular follow-up visits.

The frequency and duration of a patient's visits to a weight management program may vary depending on the out-of-pocket expenses to the patient and on the program's resources and availability. However, to ensure patient success and maximize weight loss, it is important that clinicians and patients adhere to strict follow-up schedules and timeframes. Barriers to program participation and challenges with regular attendance should be addressed prior to starting and through the weight management program.

Scheduling Considerations

Like all individuals, those seeking weight management guidance have extremely busy lives and numerous commitments, and as such, some patients may have problems finding time to participate in an intensive program. Weight management programs and their clinicians should work with each patient to devise a schedule that does not interfere with other commitments or planned activities. For example, many programs will see patients in the evenings and on weekends in order to accommodate patients who work during normal business hours or who attend school during the weekdays. Other programs will open for additional hours on holidays or offer longer days in order to accommodate patients' schedules.

The "Where" Component: Where Should a Program Take Place?

In most instances, weight management programs should take place at a centrally located healthcare clinic or facility that is easily accessible to the patient. When determining if a patient should participate in a program, the location of the program should be one of the first considerations made. Transportation to and from the facility can be a major determinant of the patient's successful completion of the program, as patients who live far away from or have difficulty getting to the program's facility may be more likely to drop out of a program.

The facility where the weight management program takes place should not only be staffed by the appropriate clinicians, but it should also be staffed by the appropriate support staff and security personnel. All staff should make a concerted effort to keep the facility clean and organized, and all spaces (e.g., offices, waiting areas) within the facility should be well-maintained and orderly.

In some cases, the patient may substitute in-person visits with telemedicine or virtual visits with their clinician. While these visits should not be the only interactions between clinician and patient, telemedicine visits do promote flexibility and may help promote compliance among patients who are unable to make frequent in-person visits.

Summary

The four components (i.e., who/what/when/where) outlined in this chapter should be included in a comprehensive weight management program. When recommending a weight management program to patients, clinicians should consider these components and make recommendations based on the program's inclusion of these components and on the program's ability to meet the patient's overall needs.

References

Academy of Nutrition and Dietetics. 2007. "Pediatric Weight Management: Executive Summary of Recommendations." www.andeal.org/topic.cfm?menu=5296&cat=3013 (accessed June 2015)

Academy of Nutrition and Dietetics. 2014. "Adult Weight Management: Executive Summary of Recommendations." www.andeal.org/topic.cfm?menu=5276&cat=4690 (accessed July 2, 2015).

American Dietetic Association. 2007. Pediatric Weight Management Evidence-Based Nutrition Practice Guideline. Chicago, IL: American Dietetic Association.

Barlow, S.E. 2007. "The Expert Committee on Child and Adolescent Overweight and Obesity of the American Academy of Pediatrics." Expert Committee Recommendations Regarding the Prevention, Assessment, and Treatment of Child and Adolescent Overweight and Obesity: Summary Report, Pediatrics 120, pp. S164–S192.

Blackwell, D.L., J.W. Lucas, and T.C. Clarke. 2014. "Summary Health Statistics for U.S. Adults: National Health Interview Survey, 2012." *Vital and Health Statistics. Series 10, Data from the National Health Survey* 10, no. 260, pp. 1–161.

Kiernan, M., S.D. Moore, D.E. Schoffman, K. Lee, A.C. King, C.B. Taylor, N.E. Kiernan, and M.G. Perri. 2012. "Social Support for Healthy Behaviors: Scale Psychometrics and Prediction of Weight Loss among Women in a Behavioral Program." *Obesity* 20, no. 4, pp. 756–64. doi:10.1038/oby.2011.293

Krebs, N.F., M.S. Jacobson, and American Academy of Pediatrics Committee on Nutrition. 2003. "Prevention of Pediatric Overweight and Obesity." *Pediatrics* 112, no. 2, pp. 424–30. doi:10.1542/peds.112.2.424

McLean, N., S. Griffin, K. Toney, and W. Hardeman. 2003. "Family Involvement in Weight Control, Weight Maintenance and Weight-Loss Interventions: A Systematic Review of Randomised Trials." *International Journal of Obesity* 27, no. 9, pp. 987–1005. doi:10.1038/sj.ijo.0802383

Ogden, C.L., M.D. Carroll, B.K. Kit, and K.M. Flegal. 2014. "Prevalence of Childhood and Adult Obesity in the United States, 2011–2012." *Jama* 311, no. 8, pp. 806–14. doi:10.1001/jama.2014.732

U.S. Department of Health and Human Services, Centers for Disease Control and Prevention. 2015. "About Child and Teen BMI." www.cdc.gov/healthyweight/assessing/bmi/childrens_bmi/about_childrens_bmi.html (accessed June 14, 2015).

Wing, R.R., and R.W. Jeffery. 1999. "Benefits of Recruiting Participants with Friends and Increasing Social Support for Weight Loss and Maintenance." *Journal of Consulting and Clinical Psychology* 67, no. 1, p. 132. doi:10.1037/0022-006x.67.1.132

CHAPTER 6

Weight Loss Intervention: Goal Setting

Once a patient has been assessed and decides to enter a weight management program, goals for achieving a healthier body weight should be set. This chapter will discuss goal setting in the context of an entire weight management program as well as from an individual patient perspective.

Overarching Goals of Weight Management Programs

Although most patients will seek weight management guidance because they (or their clinicians) dislike the number appearing on the scale, it is important that their weight not be the only goal of a weight management program. Just as health is measured a variety of ways, success in a weight management program should also be measured using more than one approach.

The first overall goal of a weight management program is curtailing weight gain and preventing future weight gain (Seagle et al. 2009, 330–46). Most individuals entering a weight management program have been slowly gaining weight over the course of several months or years; thus the first goal is to stop this trend from continuing. Many patients may not feel successful if they simply maintain their weight while in a program, but it is the clinician's duty to articulate the value in maintaining weight while establishing healthy habits.

The second, and most obvious, goal of a weight management program is the loss of body weight (Seagle et al. 2009, 330–46). Weight loss should be achievable through healthy, maintainable behaviors (i.e., without extreme dieting or restricting) and should primarily result from the loss of body fat. In order to achieve weight loss, calorie needs must be assessed and realistic caloric goals must be set. These two concepts will be discussed later in this chapter.

The third overall goal of a weight management program is improving physical and mental health (Seagle et al. 2009, 330–46). Literature has shown that a weight loss as small as 10 percent of baseline body weight can significantly improve an individual's health status (National Heart Lung and Blood Institute 1998), but health status is not solely measured by the scale. Instead, it can be measured using the multitude of assessment methods described in Chapter 4. For example, a patient who is prehypertensive may have a goal of lowering his blood pressure to 120/80. In this example, the patient's blood pressure should be taken periodically throughout the weight management program to determine success in achieving this health goal. Similar goals can be set on biochemical factors such as cholesterol and glucose levels. Mental health goals (e.g., stress reduction, feelings of increased energy) can also be measured as indicators of success in a program.

The last overall goal of a weight management program is behavior modification (Seagle et al. 2009, 330–46). Improving a patient's dietary intake and physical activity habits can produce significant weight loss, but improving those behaviors in and of themselves should also be goals of the program. Many patients will enter weight management programs having practiced poor dietary and physical activity behaviors for years or, in some cases, decades. Changing these habits is difficult. Clinicians should support all positive behavior changes by praising patients' new behaviors and reinforcing their health-promoting benefits. For example, a patient who has been losing weight quite slowly (<0.5 lb/week) but continues to consume at least 1.5 cups of fruit each day should be encouraged to continue this dietary behavior because the antioxidants and other nutrients reaped from these foods have a myriad of health benefits that may prevent future chronic diseases.

All four of these overarching goals work in concert to facilitate a high likelihood of success and provide the patient with the best experience possible.

Estimating Energy Needs

Adults

As previously discussed, the first two overarching goals of weight management are curtailing weight gain and promoting gradual weight loss. However, before the clinician can design a plan to tackle these goals, a patient's energy needs, or total energy expenditure (TEE), must be assessed. In adult patients who are overweight or obese, TEE is calculated by multiplying resting energy expenditure (REE), or resting metabolic rate, by a physical activity factor: TEE = REE × PAF.

When possible, REE should be measured using indirect calorimetry (Academy of Nutrition and Dietetics 2014). Indirect calorimetry utilizes sophisticated equipment to measure the amount of oxygen consumed and carbon dioxide produced while an individual is in a resting state. Based on these measurements, estimations of the daily REE will be made.

Although indirect calorimetry is the preferred method for obtaining REE, the necessary equipment is expensive and can be difficult to obtain. If the equipment for indirect calorimetry is not available, then the Mifflin-St. Jeor equation should be used to estimate REE for overweight and obese adults. This equation is gender-specific and takes into account a patient's height, weight, and age. The equation is found in Table 6.1.

REE estimates the number of calories an individual expends when he is at complete rest; however, most individuals are active, to some extent, throughout the day. As such, REE must be multiplied by a physical activity factor to arrive at the estimated TEE. An individual's physical activity factor can range from 1.0 to 2.4 and is based on the degree to which he is usually active. Table 6.2 lists the physical activity factors used to calculate TEE.

Table 6.1 Mifflin-St. Jeor equation for calculating REE in overweight and obese adults

Males: REE = (10 × W) + (6.25 × H) – (5 × A) + 5
Female: REE = (10 × W) + (6.25 × H) – (5 × A) – 161
W = weight in kilograms
H = height in centimeters
A = age in years

Table 6.2 Physical activity factors for calculating TEE

Sedentary: 1.0–1.3
Low active: 1.4–1.5
Active: 1.6–1.8
Very active: 1.9–2.4

Table 6.3 TEE calculations for children ages 3 to 18 years

	Boys	Girls
TEE equation*	114 – (50.9 × A) + PAF × (19.5 × W + 1,161.4 × H)	389 – (41.2 × A) + PAF × (15.0 × W + 701.6 × H)
Physical activity factors (PAF)	Sedentary: 1.00 Low active: 1.12 Active: 1.24 Very active: 1.45	Sedentary: 1.00 Low active: 1.18 Active: 1.35 Very active: 1.60

*Age (A) is measured in years. Weight (W) is measured in kilograms. Height (H) is measured in meters.

Source: Academy of Nutrition and Dietetics (2007, 11).

Children

A pediatric patient's energy needs can be estimated using methods similar to those used in adults. When possible, indirect calorimetry should be used to measure REE; however, as mentioned this is not usually feasible in a clinical setting. As such, an equation should be used to calculate TEE.

TEE equations for overweight children ages 3 to 18 years are seen in Table 6.3 (Academy of Nutrition and Dietetics 2007, 11). These equations are gender-specific and take in account the child's age, height, weight, and physical activity levels. It is important to note that the physical activity factors for children are also gender-specific.

Setting Caloric Goals

Adults

There are two recommendations on how to set an adult patient's calorie goals for weight loss. The first recommendation is to use a preestablished range of calories based on the patient's gender. For an adult female, her caloric goal would be 1,200 to 1,500 kcal/day; for an adult male, his goal would be 1,500 to 1,800 kcal/day. Using these set ranges gives patients flexibility in their diets and serves as a good starting point for weight management programs.

The second recommendation for setting caloric goals involves calculations based on the adult patient's TEE. Once a patient's TEE has been calculated, the clinician will know approximately how many calories are needed to maintain the patient at his current weight. In order to calculate the number of calories to facilitate a healthy rate of weight loss, clinicians should subtract 500 to 750 kcal from the TEE (Academy of Nutrition and Dietetics 2014). This caloric deficit should allow the patient to lose weight at a rate of 1 to 1.5 lb/week, although the actual rate may vary due to fluid fluctuations.

Box 6.1 shows a sample calculation of a patient's TEE and caloric goals for weight loss. It is often helpful to give the patient a range of calories, rather than setting a single caloric goal. In the sample calculation, a rounded range of ±10 percent the caloric goal is given to allow for flexibility in meal planning.

Box 6.1 Example calculations for TEE and setting calorie goals for weight loss

Patient: John Doe
DOB: 1/3/1952
Sex: Male
Age: 64 years
Height: 175.3 cm (69 inches)
Weight: 88.5 kg (195 lb)
Physical Activity Level: Sedentary (based on data gathered during patient interview)
Calorie Needs:

$$\text{REE} = (10 \times W) + (6.25 \times H) - (5 \times A) + 5 = (10 \times 88.5) + (6.25 \times 175.3) - (5 \times 64) + 5 = 1{,}985$$

PAL = 1.15 (mid-range of the PAL for sedentary activity)

$$\text{TEE} = \text{REE} \times \text{PAL} = 1{,}985 \times 1.15 = 2{,}283 \text{ kcal/day}$$

Calorie goals:

Goal should be 500–750 less than TEE
2,283 − 500 = 1,783 kcal/day ± 10 percent
Initial calorie goal should be set to **~1,600–1,950 kcal/day**

Because weight loss and changes in physical activity levels typically occur during weight management intervention, a patient's caloric needs and the associated caloric goals may need to be adjusted while participating in the weight management program. Caloric goals may also need to be adjusted if a patient is losing weight too quickly or too slowly. In the latter case, however, extremely low calorie diets (<1,200 kcal/day) are not recommended unless the patient is being closely supervised by a medical team.

Children

The caloric goals for pediatric patients should be based on the judgment of the Registered Dietitian Nutritionist (RDN). Because many children may not need to lose weight and, instead, may simply need to grow into their current weight, keeping their caloric intake at the current TEE and recommending additional physical activity may be sufficient. However, for those who do need to lose weight, a slight caloric deficit may be recommended. For children ages 6 to 12 years, no fewer than 900 kcal/day should be recommended, and for adolescents ages 13 to 18 years, no fewer than 1,200 kcal/day should be recommended (Academy of Nutrition and Dietetics 2007, 11). These minimum caloric intakes will ensure these children meet their nutritional needs for normal growth and development.

Establishing a Target Weight

Adults

Adults may enter weight management programs with a target weight already in mind; however, these target weights are often unrealistic and unattainable. Although the clinician should remain positive and praise the patient for seeking assistance, it is important that the clinician also ensure that the patient's weight goal is reasonable and achievable within the specified timeframe. Together, the clinician and the patient should arrive at an initial target weight, keeping in mind that once this goal is achieved, follow-up targets can be set.

Initial target weights may be set in terms of the baseline weight. As mentioned, a 10 percent loss of body weight can significantly improve an individual's health status, so this is often the first goal of a weight management program (Academy of Nutrition and Dietetics 2014). For patients with cardiovascular disease risk factors (e.g., hypertension, hyperlipidemia, and hyperglycemia), an initial weight loss of merely 3 to 5 percent can even be beneficial. This latter range can also be used when setting target weights for individuals who are heavier and further from their normal body mass index (BMI) range.

To achieve a target weight, adults should prepare for weight loss to happen at a slow and steady rate. Weight loss at a rate of up to 2 lb (or 0.9 kg)/week is appropriate for most adults (Academy of Nutrition and Dietetics 2014), and this rate is usually achievable through moderate caloric restriction and increased physical activity. The initial rate of weight loss may be higher than this recommended rate, but this rapid weight loss primarily results from the water loss associated with glycogen depletion. Once glycogen stores have been depleted, the rate of weight loss will decrease. Extended bouts of accelerated weight loss from minimal intake should generally be avoided as this may result in an excessive loss of lean body tissue (Ball, Canary, and Kyle 1967, 60–67; Benoit, Martin, and Watten 1965, 604–12) and the lowering of an individual's metabolic rate (Donnelly et al. 1991, 56–61; van Dale and Saris 1989, 409–16).

Children

Among children, target weights and rates of weight loss will depend on the child's age and on the extent of overweight or obesity. For most preschool-age children (ages 2 to 5 years), the recommendation is to simply maintain their weight while they continue to grow (Academy of Nutrition and Dietetics 2007, 11). As such, their BMI-for-age percentile will normalize to the recommended range. Only in extreme cases will weight reduction be recommended to preschool-age children, and when this does occur, the child's BMI should be greater than 21 kg/m^2 and the rate of weight loss should not exceed 1 lb/month.

For overweight children ages 6 to 12 years, the goal is also to simply maintain their weight while the child continues to grow. However, in cases where the child is obese (BMI-for-age in the 95th to 99th percentile), a slow weight loss that does not exceed 1 lb/month may be recommended. Children whose BMI is greater than the 99th percentile might also be counseled to lose weight at a rate not exceeding 2 lb/week.

During adolescence, a child's linear growth will peak, and maximum height will be reached by the end of this developmental phase. As such, the clinician should gauge where the child is in this developmental phase before establishing the child's target weight. For children early in adolescence, weight maintenance may be appropriate, as they are still growing and can potentially grow into their current weight. For overweight and obese children who have already reached or are nearing their peak height, weight loss may be prescribed. If weight loss is appropriate, a rate of no more than 2 lb/week should be recommended.

Creating Behavioral Goals to Achieve the Target Weight

Creating a target weight and sharing the desired weight loss rate with the patient are two necessary steps that should be covered at the beginning of a program. However, these steps alone are not sufficient to achieve the desired weight and health outcomes. Patients must be extensively educated on how to achieve weight loss, and goals related to these "how to" steps should be behaviorally focused.

Behavioral goals that promote weight loss are typically related to dietary intake and physical activity because those are the two primary components of energy balance. The goals, however, should not simply be "to follow the diet plan" or "to exercise more." The behavioral goals should follow the acronym, SMART, meaning they are specific, measurable, achievable, realistic, and timely (Ross et al. 2010, 327–34).

Specific behavioral goals will identify exactly what behavior the patient needs to do, as well as when and where he or she needs to do it. For example, the clinician might want his patient to practice portion control, but telling the patient to do this is too ambiguous. Instead, the clinician should develop a specific behavioral goal. In this example, asking the patient to measure the amount of cereal, sugar, and milk he puts in his bowl every morning at breakfast is much more specific and sets a clear expectation for what the patient must do.

Measurable behavioral goals will be goals that can be quantified in a meaningful way and provide insight for the patient and the clinician.

In the case of weight management, measurable goals are often ones that involve tracking. For example, the clinician can measure, or count, the number of days a patient logs what he eats in an electronic food record. If the patient's behavioral goal is to consume a total of two cups of fruit each day, then the clinician can measure the patient's success at performing this behavior by counting the number of days during which he documented consuming two cups of fruit.

Achievable and realistic behavioral goals will be behaviors that the patient can actually perform and fully reach. Although behavioral goals should be challenging and should push the patient to behave in a way outside of his current norm, the goals should never been so far-fetched that the patient will be unlikely to achieve them. This sets the patient up for frustration and failure, and it also decreases the likelihood that a patient will maintain the behavior change. Achievable, realistic goals are typically established by garnering the patient's input during the goal-setting session and by starting with small goals that are incrementally increased in behavior frequency or intensity. For example, if a patient does not normally consume breakfast, then his first behavioral goal should not be to start eating breakfast every day. Instead, the clinician should consider starting with a goal of eating breakfast on 4 days each week or every weekday. This gives the patient some flexibility when adapting to this new behavior and is a more realistic behavioral goal.

Timely behavioral goals will be behaviors, which can be accomplished in a set timeframe. When setting behavioral goals with a patient, clinicians should set a specific timeframe during which the goal should be accomplished, and in many cases the timeframe will extend from the current visit unit the follow-up appointment. Example behavioral goals that meet all of the SMART criteria are seen in Table 6.4.

Summary

While the overall goals of a weight management program should include sustainable weight loss, they should also include curbing weight gain and improving a patient's health status through behavior modification. This approach fosters a comprehensive program that will promote the development and maintenance of a healthier lifestyle.

Table 6.4 Examples of SMART behavioral goals

Goal #	What is the specific goal?	How will it be measured?	Is this goal achievable and realistic?	During what timeframe will this behavior be performed?
1	Consume 2–32 oz water bottles of water each day	Documentation on food log	Yes, because currently drinking one water bottle each day	Starting tomorrow through the follow-up visit with clinician
2	Eat a small side salad with balsamic vinegar dressing with each lunch/dinner meal in a restaurant	Documentation on food log	Yes, because only requires substituting a salad for French fries; also because usual restaurants have a salad option	Starting tonight through the follow-up visit with clinician
3	Walk on treadmill for 30 minutes at speed of 3.8 mph 5 days each week	Documentation on desk calendar	Yes, because currently walking at 3.5 mph on 3 days/week	Starting today through the follow-up visit with clinician

References

Academy of Nutrition and Dietetics. 2007. "Pediatric Weight Management: Executive Summary of Recommendations." www.andeal.org/topic.cfm?menu=5296&cat=3013 (accessed June, 2015).

Academy of Nutrition and Dietetics. 2014. "Adult Weight Management: Executive Summary of Recommendations." www.andeal.org/topic.cfm?menu=5276&cat=4690 (accessed July 2, 2015).

Ball M.F., J.J. Canary, and L.H. Kyle. 1967. "Comparative Effects of Caloric Restriction and Total Starvation on Body Composition in Obesity." *Annals of Internal Medicine* 67, no. 1, pp. 60–67. doi:10.7326/0003-4819-67-1-60

Benoit, F.L., R.L. Martin, and R.H. Watten. 1965. "Changes in Body Composition During Weight Reduction in Obesity: Balance Studies Comparing Effects of Fasting and a Ketogenic Diet." *Annals of Internal Medicine* 63, no. 4, pp. 604–12. doi:10.7326/0003-4819-63-4-604

Donnelly, J.E., N.P. Pronk, D.J. Jacobsen, S.J. Pronk, and J.M. Jakicic. 1991. "Effects of a Very-Low-Calorie Diet and Physical-Training Regimens on Body Composition and Resting Metabolic Rate in Obese Females." *The American Journal of Clinical Nutrition* 54, no. 1, pp. 56–61.

National Heart Lung and Blood Institute. 1998. Clinical Guidelines on the Identification, Evaluation, and Treatment of Overweight and Obesity in Adults [NIH Publication no. 98-4083]. National Institutes of Health. www.nhlbi.nih.gov/files/docs/guidelines/ob_gdlns.pdf

Ross, M.M., S. Kolbash, G.M. Cohen, and J.A. Skelton. 2010. "Multidisciplinary Treatment of Pediatric Obesity: Nutrition Evaluation and Management." *Nutrition in Clinical Practice: Official Publication of the American Society for Parenteral and Enteral Nutrition* 25, no. 4, pp. 327–34. doi:10.1177/0884533610373771

Seagle, H.M., G.W. Strain, A. Makris, R.S. Reeves, and American Dietetic Association. 2009. "Position of the American Dietetic Association: Weight Management." *Journal of the American Dietetic Association* 109, no. 2, pp. 330–46. doi:10.1016/j.jada.2008.11.041

van Dale, D., and W.H. Saris. 1989. "Repetitive Weight Loss and Weight Regain: Effects on Weight Reduction, Resting Metabolic Rate, and Lipolytic Activity Before and After Exercise and/or Diet Treatment." *The American Journal of Clinical Nutrition* 49, no. 3, pp. 409–16.

CHAPTER 7

Weight Loss Intervention: Energy and Macronutrient Approaches to Calorie Reduction

Weight loss programs must focus on helping patients achieve negative energy balance, but in order to do achieve this imbalance, a number of approaches can be used. In this chapter, three common approaches to adult weight management will be described, and the benefits and challenges associated with each approach will be explored. The final section will focus on macronutrient recommendations for pediatric weight management.

Very Low Calorie Diets

The paradigm of energy balance suggests that as the caloric deficit increases, so does the amount of weight lost. Therefore, an extremely low caloric intake should facilitate a fairly rapid weight loss, and this is the primary rationale for one weight loss approach, the very low calorie diet (VLCD).

VCLDs consist of fewer than 800 kcal/day (usually 500 to 800 kcal/day) and result in rapid initial weight loss, especially among those who are obese. VLCDs typically involve meal replacements, usually in the form of a liquid shake, which have been carefully formulated to help individuals following a VLCD meet a larger portion of the nutritional needs than if they were eating food alone.

Patients wanting to follow a VLCD as part of a weight loss program should only do so under the direction and close supervision of a medical team. These extreme caloric restrictions are not appropriate for all individuals, and anyone seeking to follow this kind of specialized diet should first seek a full medical evaluation.

Ingesting so few calories makes it difficult for patients to meet all of their nutritional needs. As such, a daily multivitamin with minerals may be prescribed. In addition, clinicians may want to monitor a patient's laboratory values for certain vitamins and minerals (e.g., iron, vitamin D) to ensure that the patient does not become nutrient deficient while following a VLCD.

Benefits of VLCD

In a relatively short period of time, VLCDs can produce a substantial amount of weight loss that mimics the weight loss often associated with bariatric surgery. Patients who experience this weight loss often feel a renewed sense of motivation and become encouraged by the initial weight loss. This increased motivation can spur continued compliance with the dietary restrictions, leading to further weight reduction.

In addition to weight loss, VLCDs can also assist with the rapid improvement of additional health indicators. In patients with type 2 diabetes mellitus (T2DM), VLCDs are associated with improved insulin sensitivity and β cell function (Jackness et al. 2013, 3027–32; Malandrucco et al. 2012, 609–13). VLCDs have also been associated with decreasing pericardial fat (i.e., fat accumulation around the heart, a condition associated with cardiovascular disease [CVD]) and hepatic triglyceride content (Snel et al. 2012, 1572–76), as well as improving blood pressure, inflammatory markers, and low-density lipoprotein cholesterol (Merino et al. 2013, 17–23).

Following a VLCD can also have health benefits for patients preparing to undergo weight loss surgery. One study found that patients who followed a VLCD had lower rates of postoperative complications than those who did not follow a VLCD (Van Nieuwenhove et al. 2011, 1300–305). This same study also found that surgeons perceived the surgery to be less difficult when patients follow a preoperative VLCD. In addition, another study suggested that a preoperative VLCD may reduce liver size and decrease abdominal obesity (Colles et al. 2006, 304–11). As such, some surgeons may recommend patients follow a VLCD as part of their preoperative orders.

Challenges of VLCD

Following a VLCD can result in significant weight loss, but the diet is also associated with a myriad of challenges. First and foremost is the challenge of adherence to the diet. Like most weight loss plans, VLCDs require strict adhere in order to facilitate weight loss. However, when following a VLCD, patients are not permitted to consume their typical foods, and instead, they are only allowed to consume meal replacements. This drastic shift from the patient's usual behavior can be problematic, especially when eating is associated with a social event. For example, patients may feel isolated or left out when unable to eat the same foods as their friends at certain activities and celebrations (e.g., parties and holidays). As such it is important for the patient to develop coping strategies, which will ameliorate these tempting situations.

Weight regain is also a major challenge associated with VLCDs. Because VLCDs cannot be sustained indefinitely, the patient must eventually return to eating normal foods. This transition can be difficult, especially if the patient is not receiving regular dietary guidance and support. As a result, a patient may start to regain a portion of the weight lost while following the VLCD. This tendency for weight regain is one of the reasons that some clinicians have previously advised against VLCDs (National Heart Lung and Blood Institute 1998); however, weight regain can be ameliorated by a slow reintroduction of appropriately portioned foods and by establishing new dietary habits that promote a slower rate of weight loss or weight stabilization.

Common complaints associated with following a VLCD include fatigue and tiredness. These symptoms primarily result from extreme energy restriction. Patients who report being more tired and worn-out than usual should be advised to maintain a healthy, normal sleep schedule and to perform moderate amounts of physical activity as able. In addition, patients who are prone to eat when they are tired should be monitored for these tendencies and should be advised to avoid being around food when they are fatigued.

Due to the substantial reduction in overall intake associated with a VLCD, patients may also experience constipation. When a patient eats less food, there is a reduced volume of food being passed along the gastrointestinal tract, and this can cause irregularities in bowel habits.

In addition, many of the meal replacement drinks consumed on a VLCD are low in fiber, which also increases transit time and may alter bowel habits. If constipation becomes an issue, then bulking agents, stool softeners, or fiber-containing supplements may be prescribed.

Additional side effects may be experienced by patients following a VLCD, although some of these effects are rare. Some patients have reported experiencing nausea and diarrhea when following a VLCD. The liquid meal replacement shakes are thought to contribute to these symptoms in some cases, thus warranting a change of meal replacements or an alteration of overall dietary prescription. Patients following a VLCD have also suffered more advanced medical complications, including biliary problems. One study found patients following a VLCD had a higher risk for developing gallstones than those who followed a low calorie diet (minimum of 1,200 kcal/day) (Johansson et al. 2014, 279–84). Complications and side effects of the VLCD should be carefully monitored by the attending clinician, and when necessary dietary modifications should be made to avoid adverse outcomes.

Moderate and Low-Fat Diets

By virtue of its caloric density, dietary fat has been a big target for patients (and clinicians with patients) seeking weight loss. Given that fat contains approximately 9 kcal/g, reducing dietary fat can reduce overall caloric content more than twice as much as reducing carbohydrate or protein (which have 4 kcal/g). However, low-fat and very low-fat diets have come under intense scrutiny in recent years. This scrutiny partially resulted from the insurgence of low-fat, high-sugar, high-sodium food products, which flooded the market as consumers sought to lower their fat intake as a means to eat healthier and lose weight. Because many of these products still had the same number of calories as the full-fat versions, individuals consuming these products rarely lost weight, and in some cases, ate more of the products and actually gained weight. As such, the low-fat craze has often been retrospectively viewed as a misdirection and as a contributor to the obesity epidemic.

Nevertheless, research has shown that moderate and low-fat diets can be nutritionally adequate and can facilitate weight loss if they are carefully constructed to generate a caloric deficit. For adults and children aged 4 years and older, the acceptable macronutrient distribution range (AMDR) for dietary fat is 20 to 35 percent of total calories. This translates to ~44 to 78 g of fat per day for individuals following a 2,000 kcal diet. Moderate and low-fat diets will stay within this AMDR range in order to decrease the overall caloric content of a diet, with moderate fat diets having closer to 1/3 of calories from fat and low-fat diets having closer to 20 to 25 percent of calories from fat. The AMDR ranges for 1,200, 1,500, and 1,800 kcal diets are translated into fat grams in Table 7.1.

Another fat-related characteristic of moderate and low-fat diets is the saturated fat content. Saturated fat is the type of fat commonly found in animal products and associated with increased CVD risk. As such, many health organizations recommend limiting saturated fat in all diets (weight loss and others) to no more than 10 percent of total calories. In the Dietary Approaches to Stop Hypertension (DASH), diet, arguably one of the well-researched moderate to low-fat diets, ~27 percent total calories from fat whereas only ~6 percent calories were from saturated fat (Sacks et al. 1995, 108–18). In intervention studies, the DASH diet has been shown not only to facilitate weight loss (Azadbakht et al. 2011, 55–57; Ledikwe et al. 2007, 1212–21), but it also improved blood pressure (Sacks et al. 2001, 3–10) and lipid levels (Obarzanek et al. 2001, 80–89).

Moderate or low-fat diet plans should be rich in low-calorie, nutrient-dense foods. Typically, a moderate or low-fat diet plan will include multiple servings of low-calorie fruits and vegetables in order to bulk up the volume while keeping the overall calories and fat low. Whole grains, which are typically low in fat, should be incorporated; however, the caloric density of whole grains is higher than that of most fruits and vegetables so serving sizes should be limited. Plant-based fats such as oils,

Table 7.1 Daily fat ranges for various calorie levels using AMDR of 20 to 35 percent of total calories from fat and <10 percent calories from saturated fat

Calorie level	Total fat (g/day)	Saturated fat (g/day)
1800	40–70	<20
1500	33–58	<17
1200	27–47	<13

nuts, and seeds can be incorporated in small quantities, as can foods that are prepared with these ingredients. Animal fats such as butter and lard should primarily be avoided, and the portion sizes of low-fat animal foods such as dairy and meats should be limited to keep total fat and saturated fat calories within the recommended ranges. A sample low-fat, 1,200 kcal meal plan is seen in Box 7.1, and a sample moderate fat, 1,200 kcal meal is seen in Box 7.2.

Box 7.1 Sample one-day menu for low-fat, 1,200 kcal diet

Breakfast:

1–1/2 cup dry oat-based cereal
1 cup 1% milk
1 small banana
8 oz black coffee or green tea

Lunch:

2 slices 100% whole wheat bread
1–1/2 tbsp natural peanut butter (for peanut butter sandwich)
6 oz fat-free yogurt, plain
3/4 cup blueberries (to mix into yogurt)
8 baby carrots
16 oz water

Dinner:

4 oz baked salmon
½ cup cooked quinoa
1 cup cooked broccoli
1 small orange
12 oz unsweetened ice tea

Total calories: 1213 cal
Total fat: 21% calories from total fat
Saturated fat: 4% calories from saturated fat

Box 7.2 Sample one-day menu for moderate fat, 1,200 kcal diet

Breakfast:

1 cup cooked oats
½ oz almond slivers (added to oatmeal)
½ cup 1% milk (added to oatmeal or consumed in coffee)
8 oz black coffee or green tea

Lunch:

2 cups garden salad with lettuce, tomatoes, and carrots
4 slices of avocado (to add to the salad)
2 oz skinless or boneless grilled chicken breast (to add to the salad)
2 tbsps oil and vinegar dress (to add to the salad)
1 medium apple
1 cup skim milk

Dinner:

½ cup brown rice
1 cup steamed green beans
1 medium pork chop, lean
8 oz light vanilla yogurt
¾ cup blackberries (to add to yogurt)
16 oz water

Total calories: 1209 cal
Total fat: 31% calories from fat
Saturated fat: 6% calories from saturated fat

Benefits of Moderate and Low-Fat Diets

As long as an energy deficit is created, moderate and low-fat diets can produce weight loss at the same rate as other energy-restricted diets. Because fat is the primary restriction, these diets can be high in nutrient-dense, carbohydrate-containing foods, and they can provide a nutritionally adequate diet. For example, most fruits and vegetables are naturally low in fat (the exception being avocado), yet they are high in vitamins, minerals, and antioxidants. As such, moderate and low-fat diets that contain high amounts of fresh or minimally processed fruits and vegetables also tend to be low in calories and able to facilitate weight loss.

Because moderate and low-fat diets tend to be high in fruits and vegetables, they also tend to be high in fiber. Fiber is one of the plant-based nutrients found in high quantities in fruits and vegetables. Fiber promotes satiety as well as overall gastrointestinal health and bowel regularity. Fiber can also be found in whole grains, which are another component of the moderate and low-fat diet. Whole grains are also naturally low in fat; however, patients must limit the portion sizes of whole grains and other starch-based plant foods (e.g., potatoes and corn) as they are more calorically dense than most nonstarchy vegetables and fruits.

A moderate and low-fat diet has also been shown to lower the risk of CVD in adults (Junker et al. 2001, 355–66; Marckmann, Sandstrom, and Jespersen 1994, 935–39). In particular, the low amount of saturated fat recommended in a moderate or low-fat diet has also been associated with lowering the risk of CVD (Eckel et al. 2014, 2960–84). Given that obese patients typically exhibit one or more CVD risk factors (e.g., elevated blood pressure and cholesterol), it is often advantageous to seek out diets such as the moderate and low-fat diet that also promote heart health in order to improve these other risk factors.

The primary sources of fat in a moderate and low-fat diet will be monounsaturated and polyunsaturated fats. Among the polyunsaturated fats, linoleic acid (n-6 fatty acids) and α-linolenic acid (n-3 fatty acids) are two essential fatty acids, which must be ingested because humans do not possess the ability to synthesize them in the body. Moderate and low-fat diets should be carefully created to achieve adequate intakes of these two fatty acids. The Institute of Medicine, currently recommends that 5 to 10 percent of total calories come from linoleic acid and 0.6 to 1.2 percent of total calories come from α-linolenic acid (Institute of Medicine 2005).

Challenges of Moderate and Low-Fat Diets

Just because a diet plan is moderate or low in fat does not necessarily mean that it will produce weight loss. In order to produce weight loss, the diet plan must create a caloric deficit. As such, total caloric intake must remain controlled and restricted even when following a moderate or low-fat diet.

Often times, patients following a moderate or low-fat diet will mistakenly think that all low-fat food products (e.g., low-fat cookies and snack foods) are good alternatives to the full-fat versions. As mentioned previously, these modified products are often just as high in calories as the full-fat versions because the fat has been replaced by other calorie-containing ingredients such as sugar or starch. Because this is an easy mistake to make, it is important that clinicians help patients learn to read nutrition labels and help them to identify what low-fat foods are appropriate and inappropriate to consume when following a low-fat diet.

Another challenge associated with moderate and low-fat diets is the concept of healthy versus less healthy fats. Foods containing the healthier fats (e.g., olive oil, nuts, avocado, and fish that contain monounsaturated and polyunsaturated fats) should be incorporated into a moderate and low-fat diet in order to maintain nutritional adequacy. However, the portion sizes of foods containing healthy fats should be limited because, like any fat-containing food, they can be quite calorically dense. Patients often have the misconception that healthy fats can be consumed in unrestricted amounts, but the truth is that these foods can have just as many (or sometimes more) calories than foods containing less healthy fats. It is up to the clinician to ensure patients understand how portion control must be exercised when consuming sources of healthy fats.

Low-Carbohydrate Diets

When it comes to the three essential macronutrients (carbohydrate, fat, and protein), fat has traditionally been the target for weight reduction strategies because of its high energy density. However, mounting evidence also supports the effectiveness of a low-carbohydrate diet in producing weight loss, and many clinicians and patients now utilize this strategy as an initial and long-term means to cut calories and reduce body weight.

Over the past several decades, research has demonstrated that carbohydrate-restricted diets can produce weight loss at a rate that is similar to (Clifton, Condo, and Keogh 2014, 224–35; Dutton, Laitner, and Perri 2014, 1–14; Naude et al. 2014), or in some cases even greater than (Bueno et al. 2013, 1178–87) weight loss achieved by other reduced calorie diets. As a result, many health and professional organizations now promote a variety of dietary approaches, including carbohydrate-restricted diets, as a means to achieving weight loss goals.

For adults and children aged 1 year and older, the Recommended Dietary Allowance of carbohydrates is 130 g each day, or 45–65 percent of total calories (Institute of Medicine 2005). However, these levels are higher than those recommended in a low-carbohydrate diet. In low-carbohydrate diets, carbohydrate intake is restricted to 20–60 g/day (Last and Wilson 2006, 1951–58), and in very low-carbohydrate diets, the amount of carbohydrate is further restricted to <20 g/day (Brinkworth et al. 2009, 23–32).

By limiting carbohydrate intake, body weight is lost through several mechanisms. Initial weight loss, which can be rapid and dramatic, is primarily due to the diuretic effect of glycogen depletion. Glycogen stores in the body become depleted because there is minimal blood glucose to use as fuel, and glycogen is used as fuel instead. As the body burns through its glycogen stores, water is released, and water weight is lost. Seeing this rapid and dramatic decrease in the number on the scale can serve as a great motivator to some patients, especially at the beginning of a weight loss program. However, it should be noted that this water weight is typically regained as soon as normal amounts of carbohydrates are reintroduced in the diet.

In low-carbohydrate diets, weight loss also occurs as the body transitions into a state of ketosis. Ketosis occurs when inadequate amounts of carbohydrates are ingested and low levels of blood glucose and insulin are experienced. Low levels of glucose and insulin stimulate the breakdown of adipose tissue, and from this breakdown, ketone bodies are formed. The ketone bodies can then be used as a source of fuel for the brain, and in this ketogenic state, hunger may also be depressed (Johnstone et al. 2008, 44–55).

The presence of ketones, which can be measured using urinary ketone detection strips, is often considered a highly desirable state as it is an indication that the body is breaking down adipose tissue or fat mass. In some short-term studies, low-carbohydrate diets have resulted in greater reductions in fat mass than other isocaloric diets (Brehm et al. 2003, 1617–23; Volek et al. 2004, 13), and in some interventions, low-carbohydrate diets have also been shown to improve lipid profiles and reduce the risk of metabolic syndrome (Volek, Sharman, and Forsythe 2005, 1339–42).

Although the body does break down fat while in the ketogenic state, it also breaks down lean body tissue and muscle mass. This is a major concern to most clinicians, so to mitigate this, physical activity and exercise are highly recommended as part of the weight management program. In particular, resistance training has been shown to promote a reduction in fat mass while retaining lean body mass (Jabekk et al. 2010, 17).

Benefits of Low-Carbohydrate Diets

Many patients will prefer to follow a low-carbohydrate diet over other types of diets because they may require less planning and, to some extent, less portion control. The primary focus of low-carbohydrate diets is on limiting the total amount of carbohydrates ingested, and by sheer virtue of limiting carbohydrates, most individuals will inadvertently lower their total caloric intake. This results in negative energy balance and a resultant weight loss.

Because the low-carbohydrate diet eliminates consumption of most starchy and sugary foods, individuals following this diet will be more likely to have very low intakes of empty-calorie foods. Savory snack foods such as potato chips, pretzels, and flavored crisps and crackers are not permitted on the low-carbohydrate diet, and sugary treats such as cakes, candies and candy bars, and cookies are also prohibited. In a typical diet, these foods contribute little, if any, nutritional value, so by eliminating them as part of the low-carbohydrate diet, there is minimal health consequence. Eliminating these foods can also help patients break the habit of unhealthy snacking, another positive side effect of this kind of diet.

Another benefit to following a low-carbohydrate diet is that it does promote the inclusion of a wide variety of nonstarchy, low-calorie vegetables. Consuming these vegetables at every meal should help the patient to meet his vitamin and mineral needs, especially those of vitamin A, vitamin C, and potassium. The sample menu in Box 7.3 demonstrates how these low-calorie vegetables can be incorporated at all three meals.

Box 7.3 Example of a low-carbohydrate, 1,200 kcal diet

Breakfast:

2 whole eggs scrambled with tomato, onion, and green pepper
1 oz cheddar cheese (added to scrambled eggs)
2 slices avocado (added to scrambled egg)
8 oz black coffee or green tea

Lunch:

4 cups of grilled chicken salad (includes grilled chicken, bacon, lettuce, cheese, tomatoes, and carrots)
3 tbsps Italian dressing
12 oz unsweetened iced tea

Dinner:

4 oz grilled steak, lean
1 cup cooked collard and mustard greens
1 cup fat-free Greek yogurt, plain
1 cup whole strawberries
16 oz water

Total calories: 1,194 kcal
Total carbohydrates: 44 g, 15% calories from carbohydrate

Challenges of Low-Carbohydrate Diets

The main challenge associated with low-carbohydrate and very low-carbohydrate diets is the restrictive nature of these diets. Most readily available foods, both healthy and not-so-healthy, contain some amount of carbohydrates. For example, fruits, with their myriad of antioxidants and phytochemicals, are almost entirely composed of carbohydrate. For individuals following a low-carbohydrate diet, these otherwise healthy foods must be limited and avoided in order to keep total carbohydrate intake low. This notion of limiting intake of health-promoting foods can be confusing to some patients.

To reduce confusion and promote healthier eating behaviors, clinicians may find it helpful to give the patient a list of lower carbohydrate plant-based foods in order to ensure that the patient still receives the benefits of a plant-based diet. Box 7.4 includes a list of lower carbohydrate plant-based foods as well as their serving sizes and carbohydrate contents. It is important to remember that higher carbohydrate foods can be incorporated into a low-carbohydrate diet as long as their portions are controlled and their carbohydrate content is incorporated into the daily allotment of carbohydrates.

Box 7.4 Example of lower carbohydrate plant-based foods that can be incorporated into low-carbohydrate diets

Fruits:

- Blackberries (3/4 cup = 10 g carbohydrate)
- Blueberries (1/2 cup = 11 g carbohydrate)
- Cantaloupe (1 medium wedge from medium melon = 6 g carbohydrate)
- Casaba melon (1 cup = 11 g carbohydrate)
- Clementine (1 small Clementine = 10 g carbohydrate)
- Grapefruit (1/2 medium grapefruit = 10 g carbohydrate)
- Honeydew (1 medium wedge = 11 g carbohydrate)
- Raspberries (3/4 cup = 11 g carbohydrate)
- Strawberries (1 cup whole = 11 g carbohydrate)
- Watermelon (10 watermelon balls = 9 g carbohydrate)

Vegetables:

- Asparagus (7 medium spears = 5 g carbohydrate)
- Avocado (4 slices = 3 g carbohydrate)
- Broccoli (1 cup, raw, chopped = 6 g carbohydrate)
- Brussel sprouts (1 cup, cooked = 11 g carbohydrate)
- Cactus (1 cup, raw = 5 g carbohydrate)

(*Continued*)

(*Continued*)

Cauliflower (1 cup, raw = 5 g carbohydrate)
Collard greens (1 cup cooked = 10 g carbohydrate)
Cucumber (1 large = 6 g carbohydrate)
Green beans (1 cup, cooked = 11 g carbohydrate)
Green pepper (1 large pepper = 8 g carbohydrate)
Jalapeno pepper (5 peppers = 6 g carbohydrate)
Jicama (1 cup = 11 g carbohydrate)
Kale (1 cup cooked = 7 g carbohydrate)
Lettuce (2 cups iceberg or mixed greens = 3 g carbohydrate)
Okra (1 cup cooked = 10 g carbohydrate)
Onion (1/2 cup, chopped, raw = 7 g carbohydrate)
Spaghetti squash (1 cup cooked = 10 g carbohydrate)
Spinach (2 cups raw = 2 g carbohydrate)
Summer squash (1 medium, yellow, raw = 7 g carbohydrate)
Tomato (1 medium whole tomato = 5 g carbohydrate)
Zucchini (1 medium, green, raw = 6 g carbohydrate)

Legumes and grains:

Black beans (1/4 cup cooked = 10 g carbohydrate)
Black-eyed peas (1/3 cup cooked = 11 g carbohydrate)
Hummus (3 tbsps = 9 g carbohydrate)
Kidney beans (1/4 cup cooked = 9 g carbohydrate)
Lentils (1/4 cup cooked = 10 g carbohydrate)
Lima beans (1/4 cup cooked = 9 g carbohydrate)
Oatmeal (1/3 cup cooked = 9 g carbohydrate)
Pinto beans (1/4 cup cooked = 11 g carbohydrate)
Quinoa (1/3 cup cooked = 12 g carbohydrate)
Soybeans (1/2 cup cooked = 9 g carbohydrate)
Whole-wheat bread, reduced calorie (1 small slice = 10 g carbohydrate)

Source: U.S. Department of Agriculture, Agriculture Research Service, What's in the Foods You Eat Search Tool. www.ars.usda.gov/Services/docs.htm?docid=17032

Because of the limited amount of plant-based foods, which can be incorporated into a low-carbohydrate diet, patients following these diets may find it difficult to meet their daily fiber needs. This can result in constipation and irregularities in bowel function, which can be frustrating and troublesome. In order to resolve this issue, clinicians should help patients incorporate as many high-fiber, low-carbohydrate vegetables as they can into their meal plan, with a goal of consuming at least 25 g of fiber a day (the adequate intake levels for most adult females [Institute of Medicine 2005]).

Low-carbohydrate diets may not be appropriate for all patient populations. For example, clinicians should use caution when advising young children and athletes to follow carbohydrate-restricted diets as these individuals may have higher carbohydrate needs given their life stages and activity levels. In addition, low-carbohydrate diets may be appropriate for all patients with diabetes (T1DM or T2DM). If advised to follow such a diet, these patients should be closely monitored by a healthcare clinician. Although studies have shown that low-carbohydrate diets can improve glycemic control (Yancy et al. 2005, 34), a carbohydate-restricted diet may be contraindicated in patients taking certain diabetes medications because of the risk for hypoglycemia.

Macronutrient Distribution for Pediatric Weight Management

Unlike adults, overweight and obese children are still experiencing periods of growth and development. Because their bodies are undergoing these changes, it is essential that their nutrient needs be met, even while following a weight loss regimen. As such, most clinicians will keep these young patients' dietary prescriptions within the AMDRs for carbohydrates, fat, and protein (shown in Box 7.5), and avoid excessive restrictions of certain macronutrient-dense foods.

Box 7.5 AMDRs for children and adolescents

Carbohydrates:

2–18 years: 45%–65% of total calories

Total fat:

2–3 years: 30%–40% of total calories

(*Continued*)

(*Continued*)

4–18 years: 25%–35% of total calories
Protein:
2–3 years: 5%–20% of total calories
4–18 years: 10%–30% of total calories

Source: Institute of Medicine (2005).

According to the Academy of Nutrition and Dietetics, there are some instances in which a modified diet may be appropriate for pediatric weight loss (Academy of Nutrition and Dietetics 2007, 11). A low-carbohydrate diet (20 to 60 g carbohydrate diet) may be recommended to some adolescents for short periods of time (up to 12 weeks). Similarly, a protein-sparing modified fast may be recommended to children or adolescents who are >20 percent above their ideal body weight, have serious medical conditions, and if they would benefit from rapid weight loss. However, this modified fast should not be recommended for >10 weeks and should only be followed while under close medical supervision. Very low-fat diets (<20 percent of total calories) should never be recommended as a weight management strategy for children or adolescents.

Summary

Because they all can result in negative energy balance, VLCDs, moderate and low-fat diets, and low-carbohydrate diets have all been shown to facilitate short- and long-term weight loss in overweight and obese adults. As a result, any of these approaches can be utilized as part of a reduced calorie diet plan to help adult patients achieve their long-term weight-related goals. When working with pediatric patients, however, a more moderate dietary approach should be utilized, and over-restriction of certain macronutrients should only be used in certain cases.

References

Academy of Nutrition and Dietetics. 2007. "Pediatric Weight Management: Executive Summary of Recommendations." www.andeal.org/topic.cfm?menu=5296&cat=3013 (accessed June, 2015).

Azadbakht, L., N.R. Fard, M. Karimi, M.H. Baghaei, P.J. Surkan, M. Rahimi, A. Esmaillzadeh, and W.C. Willett. 2011. "Effects of the Dietary Approaches to Stop Hypertension (DASH) Eating Plan on Cardiovascular Risks Among Type 2 Diabetic Patients: A Randomized Crossover Clinical Trial." *Diabetes Care* 34, no. 1, pp. 55–57. doi:10.2337/dc10-0676

Brehm, B.J., R.J. Seeley, S.R. Daniels, and D.A. D'Alessio. 2003. "A Randomized Trial Comparing a Very Low Carbohydrate Diet and a Calorie-Restricted Low Fat Diet on Body Weight and Cardiovascular Risk Factors in Healthy Women." *The Journal of Clinical Endocrinology and Metabolism* 88, no. 4, pp. 1617–23. doi:10.1210/jc.2002-021480

Brinkworth, G.D., M. Noakes, J.D. Buckley, J.B. Keogh, and P.M. Clifton. 2009. "Long-Term Effects of a Very-Low-Carbohydrate Weight Loss Diet Compared with an Isocaloric Low-Fat Diet After 12 Mo." *The American Journal of Clinical Nutrition* 90, no. 1, pp. 23–32. doi:10.3945/ajcn.2008.27326

Bueno, N.B., I.S.V. de Melo, S.L. de Oliveira, and T. da Rocha Ataide. 2013. "Very-Low-Carbohydrate Ketogenic Diet v. Low-Fat Diet for Long-Term Weight Loss: A Meta-Analysis of Randomised Controlled Trials." *British Journal of Nutrition* 110, no. 7, pp. 1178–87. doi:10.1017/S0007114513000548

Clifton, P.M., D. Condo, and J.B. Keogh. 2014. "Long Term Weight Maintenance After Advice to Consume Low Carbohydrate, Higher Protein Diets–A Systematic Review and Meta Analysis." *Nutrition, Metabolism and Cardiovascular Diseases* 24, no. 3, pp. 224–35. doi:10.1016/j.numecd.2013.11.006

Colles, S.L., J.B. Dixon, P. Marks, B.J. Strauss, and P.E. O'Brien. 2006. "Preoperative Weight Loss with a Very-Low-Energy Diet: Quantitation of Changes in Liver and Abdominal Fat by Serial Imaging." *The American Journal of Clinical Nutrition* 84, no. 2, pp. 304–11.

Dutton, G.R., M.H. Laitner, and M.G. Perri. 2014. "Lifestyle Interventions for Cardiovascular Disease Risk Reduction: A Systematic Review of the Effects of Diet Composition, Food Provision, and Treatment Modality on Weight Loss." *Current Atherosclerosis Reports* 16, no. 10, pp. 1–14. doi:10.1007/s11883-014-0442-0

Eckel, R.H., J.M. Jakicic, J.D. Ard, J.M. de Jesus, N. Houston Miller, V.S. Hubbard, I.M. Lee, A.H. Lichtenstein, C.M. Loria, B.E. Millen, C.A. Nonas, F.M. Sacks, S.C. Smith, L.P. Svetkey, T.A. Wadden, and S.Z. Yanovski. 2014. "2013 AHA/ACC Guideline on Lifestyle Management to Reduce Cardiovascular Risk: A Report of the American College of Cardiology/American Heart Association Task Force on Practice Guidelines." *Journal of the American College of Cardiology* 63, no. 25_PA, pp. 2960–84. doi:10.1016/j.jacc.2013.11.003

Institute of Medicine. 2005. "Table: Dietary Reference Intakes Values Summary." http://iom.nationalacademies.org/~/media/Files/Activity%20Files/Nutrition/DRIs/5_Summary%20Table%20Tables%201-4.pdf (accessed June 18, 2015).

Jabekk, P.T., I.A. Moe, H.D. Meen, S.E. Tomten, and A.T. Høstmark. 2010. "Resistance Training in Overweight Women on a Ketogenic Diet Conserved Lean Body Mass while Reducing Body Fat." *Nutrition and Metabolism (London)* 7, p. 17. doi:10.1186/1743-7075-7-17

Jackness, C., W. Karmally, G. Febres, I.M. Conwell, L. Ahmed, M. Bessler, D.J. McMahon, and J. Korner. 2013. "Very Low-Calorie Diet Mimics the Early Beneficial Effect of Roux-En-Y Gastric Bypass on Insulin Sensitivity and Beta-Cell Function in Type 2 Diabetic Patients." *Diabetes* 62, no. 9, pp. 3027–32. doi:10.2337/db12-1762

Johansson, K., J. Sundström, C. Marcus, E. Hemmingsson, and M. Neovius. 2014. "Risk of Symptomatic Gallstones and Cholecystectomy After a Very-Low-Calorie Diet or Low-Calorie Diet in a Commercial Weight Loss Program: 1-Year Matched Cohort Study." *International Journal of Obesity* 38, no. 2, pp. 279–84. doi:10.1038/ijo.2013.83

Johnstone, A.M., G.W. Horgan, S.D. Murison, D.M. Bremner, and G.E. Lobley. 2008. "Effects of a High-Protein Ketogenic Diet on Hunger, Appetite, and Weight Loss in Obese Men Feeding Ad Libitum." *The American Journal of Clinical Nutrition* 87, no. 1, pp. 44–55.

Junker, R., B. Pieke, H. Schulte, R. Nofer, M. Neufeld, G. Assmann, and U. Wahrburg. 2001. "Changes in Hemostasis During Treatment of Hypertriglyceridemia With a Diet Rich in Monounsaturated and n-3 Polyunsaturated Fatty Acids in Comparison with a Low-Fat Diet." *Thrombosis Research* 101, no. 5, pp. 355–66. doi:10.1016/s0049-3848(00)00421-7

Last, A.R., and S.A. Wilson. 2006. "Low-Carbohydrate Diets." *American Family Physician* 73, no. 11, pp. 1951–58.

Ledikwe, J.H., B.J. Rolls, H. Smiciklas-Wright, D.C. Mitchell, J.D. Ard, C. Champagne, N. Karanja, P.H. Lin, V.J. Stevens, and L.J. Appel. 2007. "Reductions in Dietary Energy Density Are Associated with Weight Loss in Overweight and Obese Participants in the PREMIER Trial." *The American Journal of Clinical Nutrition* 85, no. 5, pp. 1212–21.

Malandrucco, I., P. Pasqualetti, I. Giordani, D. Manfellotto, F. De Marco, F. Alegiani, A.M. Sidoti, F. Picconi, A. Di Flaviani, G. Frajese, R.C. Bonadonna, and S. Frontoni. 2012. "Very-Low-Calorie Diet: A Quick Therapeutic Tool to Improve Beta Cell Function in Morbidly Obese Patients with Type 2 Diabetes." *The American Journal of Clinical Nutrition* 95, no. 3, pp. 609–13. doi:10.3945/ajcn.111.023697

Marckmann, P., B. Sandstrom, and J. Jespersen. 1994. "Low-Fat, High-Fiber Diet Favorably Affects Several Independent Risk Markers of Ischemic Heart Disease: Observations on Blood Lipids, Coagulation, and Fibrinolysis from a Trial of Middle-Aged Danes." *The American Journal of Clinical Nutrition* 59, no. 4, pp. 935–39.

Merino, J., I. Megias-Rangil, R. Ferré, N. Plana, J. Girona, A. Rabasa, G. Aragonés, A. Cabré, A. Bonada, and M. Heras. 2013. "Body Weight Loss by Very-Low-Calorie Diet Program Improves Small Artery Reactive Hyperemia in Severely Obese Patients." *Obesity Surgery* 23, no. 1, pp. 17–23. doi:10.1007/s11695-012-0729-6

National Heart Lung and Blood Institute. 1998. Clinical Guidelines on the Identification, Evaluation, and Treatment of Overweight and Obesity in Adults [NIH Publication no. 98-4083]. National Institutes of Health.

Naude, C.E., A. Schoonees, M. Senekal, T. Young, P. Garner, and J. Volmink. 2014. "Low Carbohydrate Versus Isoenergetic Balanced Diets for Reducing Weight and Cardiovascular Risk: A Systematic Review and Meta-Analysis." *PLoS ONE* 9, no. 7: e100652. doi:10.1371/journal.pone.0100652

Obarzanek, E., F.M. Sacks, W.M. Vollmer, G.A. Bray, E.R. Miller 3rd, P.H. Lin, N.M. Karanja, M.M. Most-Windhauser, T.J. Moore, J.F. Swain, C.W. Bales, M.A. Proschan, and on behalf of the DASH Research Group. 2001. "Effects on Blood Lipids of a Blood Pressure-Lowering Diet: The Dietary Approaches to Stop Hypertension (DASH) Trial." *The American Journal of Clinical Nutrition* 74, no. 1, pp. 80–89.

Sacks, F.M., E. Obarzanek, M.M. Windhauser, L.P. Svetkey, W.M. Vollmer, M. McCullough, N. Karanja, P.H. Lin, P. Steele, M.A. Proschan, M.A. Evans, L.J. Appel, G.A. Bray, T.M. Vogt, T.J. Moore, and DASH Investigators. 1995. "Rationale and Design of the Dietary Approaches to Stop Hypertension Trial (DASH): A Multicenter Controlled-Feeding Study of Dietary Patterns to Lower Blood Pressure." *Annals of Epidemiology* 5, no. 2, pp. 108–18. doi:10.1016/1047-2797(94)00055-x

Sacks, F.M., L.P. Svetkey, W.M. Vollmer, L.J. Appel, G.A. Bray, D. Harsha, E. Obarzanek, P.R. Conlin, E.R. Miller, and D.G. Simons-Morton. 2001. "Effects on Blood Pressure of Reduced Dietary Sodium and the Dietary Approaches to Stop Hypertension (DASH) Diet." *New England Journal of Medicine* 344, no. 1, pp. 3–10. doi:10.1056/nejm200101043440101

Snel, M, J.T. Jonker, S. Hammer, G. Kerpershoek, H.J. Lamb, A. Meinders, H. Pijl, A. Roos, J.A. Romijn, J.W.A. Smit, and I.M. Jazet. 2012. "Long-Term Beneficial Effect of a 16-Week Very Low Calorie Diet on Pericardial Fat in Obese Type 2 Diabetes Mellitus Patients." *Obesity* 20, no. 8, pp. 1572–76. doi:10.1038/oby.2011.390

Van Nieuwenhove, Y., Z. Dambrauskas, A. Campillo-Soto, F. Van Dielen, R. Wiezer, I. Janssen, M. Kramer, and A. Thorell. 2011. "Preoperative Very Low-Calorie Diet and Operative Outcome After Laparoscopic Gastric Bypass: A Randomized Multicenter Study." *Archives of Surgery* 146, no. 11, pp. 1300–305. doi:10.1001/archsurg.2011.273

Volek, J., M. Sharman, A. Gomez, D.A. Judelson, M.R. Rubin, G. Watson, B. Sokmen, R. Silvestre, D.N. French, and W.J. Kraemer. 2004. "Comparison of Energy-Restricted Very Low-Carbohydrate and Low-Fat Diets on Weight Loss and Body Composition in Overweight Men and Women." *Nutrition and Metabolism (London)* 1, no. 1, p. 13.

Volek, J.S., M.J. Sharman, and C.E. Forsythe. 2005. "Modification of Lipoproteins by Very Low-Carbohydrate Diets." *The Journal of Nutrition* 135, no. 6, pp. 1339–42.

Yancy, W.S., Jr., M. Foy, A.M. Chalecki, M.C. Vernon, and E.C. Westman. 2005. "A Low-Carbohydrate, Ketogenic Diet to Treat Type 2 Diabetes." *Nutrition and Metabolism* 2, p. 34. doi: 10.1186/1743-7075-2-34

CHAPTER 8

Weight Loss Intervention: Basic Concepts for Nutrition Education

Without basic nutrition knowledge, an individual may struggle to effectively manage his weight. As such, it is imperative that key concepts be conveyed through basic nutrition education as part of a comprehensive weight management program. This chapter will explore some of these key concepts and will also provide examples on how these concepts can be incorporated into the program.

Empty Calorie Foods

In a comprehensive weight management program, one of the most basic concepts that should be conveyed during the first nutrition education session is the concept of empty calories and empty calorie foods. Empty calories are essentially the calories contributed by solid fats and added sugars, which add little to no nutritional value to the diet. Empty calorie foods are calorie-containing foods and beverages, which tend to be high in solid fats and added sugars, and have few nutrients, antioxidants, or phytochemicals. In essence, the calories consumed from these foods are not nutrient-dense and, therefore, provide minimal health benefit.

Because individuals seeking weight management will need to limit the number of calories they consume, they will need to ensure that all of the foods and beverages they eat are as nutrient-dense as possible; therefore, they should limit the number of empty calories and empty calorie foods they eat and drink on a daily basis.

Some examples of empty calorie foods are seen in Box 8.1. Although these foods and beverages should be avoided most of the time, they may be incorporated into meal plans on special occasions. When consuming empty calorie foods, the portions of other foods must be reduced if the patient wants to maintain a caloric deficit.

Box 8.1 ***Examples of empty calorie foods***

Foods:

- Cheese-flavored puffs or chips
- Cookies
- Cakes
- Donuts and pastries
- Potato chips or flavored crisps
- Sugary cereals
- Unfortified, refined grain products

Beverages:

- Fruit-flavored drinks (e.g., fruit punch)
- Sugar-sweetened sodas
- Sugar-sweetened energy drinks

The concept of empty calories and empty calorie foods can be taught using a variety of methods. In Box 8.2, an example exercise is outlined wherein the instructor uses teaspoons to measure the amount of sugar (i.e., empty calories) which are present in a 2 L soda.

Box 8.2 ***Instructional ideas for teaching the concept of empty calories***

What you need:

- Teaspoon
- Sugar
- 2 L bottle of regular (non-diet) cola
- Zipper-sealed bag

Instructions:

1. Explain to the patient what empty calories and empty calorie foods are.

2. Show the patient the sugar, and explain that added sugars are considered empty calories.
3. Multiply the grams of sugars (from the nutrition facts label) by the number of servings in the 2 L bottle (e.g., 27 g × 8 servings per 2 L bottle = 216 g) to get the total grams of sugar in a 2 L bottle.
4. Divide the total grams of sugar by 4 (e.g., 216/4 g = 54 tsp) to get the number of teaspoons of sugar in a 2 L bottle.
5. Ask the patient to measure out 54 tsp of sugar and place it into the zipper-sealed bag. This bag will then give a visual representation how many empty calories are in a 2 L bottle of regular cola.

Portion Control

The second concept that should be introduced early in a weight management program is the concept of portion control. This concept is critical to weight management success because it helps the patient to understand how much food he can eat in order to maintain a caloric deficit.

Because the portion sizes of most foods and beverages sold on the market are much larger than a single serving, many patients will need to be educated on what an appropriate serving size or portion looks like. Appropriate portion sizes will vary depending on the caloric content of the food. For example, nonstarchy vegetables have fewer calories than starchy vegetables; thus an appropriate portion size of fresh spinach will usually be larger than that of steamed corn.

To help control portion sizes and, in turn, control caloric intake, patients should be encouraged to measure the amount of food they serve themselves at home. Many patients will control portions by serving foods with measuring cups, teaspoons, and tablespoons. For example, a patient might use a 1/3-cup measuring cup to serve brown rice (i.e., an 80 kcal portion) and use a tablespoon to measure dressing for their salad (i.e., a ~45 kcal portion for oil-based dressings). Using these measuring utensils will help the patient to more easily identify appropriate portion sizes. In addition, when these exact portions are documented on a food log, it will also help the clinician analyze exactly how many calories and nutrients the patient is ingesting.

Patients can also control the portion sizes of foods consumed at home by using smaller plates, bowls, and glasses. Over the past three decades, the average size of a plate has grown 2 inches in diameter and 44 percent in the surface area (Klara 2004, 14–15), thus making room for more food and more calories. As such, patients should be encouraged to use the smallest plates, bowls, and glasses they can find in order to help limit the amount of calories they consume at a sitting. For example, instead of eating cereal from a large bowl, a patient could use a small sundae bowl or even a coffee mug.

Another strategy for controlling portions is the use of the plate method (Camelon et al. 1998, 1155–58). In this strategy, patients do not necessarily have to measure their foods; however, they do have to ensure that they consume their meals from a plate and that the plate is correctly divided into the various food groups. Using the plate method, one-half of the plate should contain nonstarchy vegetables, one-quarter of the plate should contain grains (ideally, whole grains) or starchy vegetables, and one-quarter of the plate should contain a source of protein (ideally, lean protein). A small serving of fruit or low-fat dairy may also be served on the side of the plate. A visual of the plate method is seen in Figure 8.1.

Meals served in restaurants are often calorie-laden and detrimental to those who are trying to lose weight. It is especially important to encourage weight management patients to limit the number of large meals

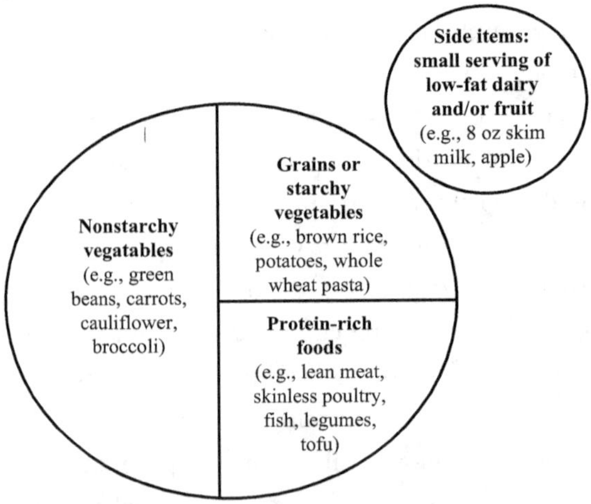

Figure 8.1 Example of the plate method

Source: Adapted from Camelon et al., 1998.

they consume in restaurant establishments. However, given that foods prepared away from the home account for >40 percent of adults' food expenditures and nearly one-third of calories consumed (Lin and Guthrie 2012), it is important to teach patients how to eat the right portion sizes when they are eating foods prepared outside the home.

Strategies for portion control when eating out include, but are not limited to:

- Order off the kids or senior citizen's menu (these portion sizes tend to be smaller and lower in calories than options on the regular menu)
- Ask for half of the meal to be placed in a to-go container prior to it being served (this will ensure that only half of the meal is consumed at the one sitting, and the other half can be eaten at a later time)
- Order a side salad with a low-calorie dressing or a broth-based soup (these appetizers are low-calorie and filling, and by eating them, the patient may be less likely to consume a large main entrée)
- Ask for chips, bread, and breadsticks to be served with the main entrée (this will prevent the patient from filling up on these high-calorie items before the main entrée is served)
- Avoid ordering calorie-containing beverages; order water, unsweetened tea or coffee, or seltzer water
- Avoid ordering an appetizer or dessert for one person; always split these items between multiple people
- Use the plate method when dining at buffets, and only allow one trip to the buffet line

Reading Nutrition Facts Labels

An enormous amount of relevant information can be gleaned by reading nutrition facts labels, and studies have shown that those who read labels consume less fat (Neuhouser, Kristal, and Patterson 1999, 45–53) and fewer calories (Temple et al. 2011, S52–55) than those who do not. As such, when a patient begins a weight management program, he should immediately be instructed on how to read and use the information on nutrition facts labels.

When initially teaching patients how to read nutrition facts labels, the clinician should emphasize the serving size before he teaches anything else. The first thing an individual should do when he reads a nutrition facts label is identify the serving size of that product. All of the information on the nutrition facts panel pertains to that one serving size, even if the entire package contains multiple servings. The serving size is key to understanding how many calories and other nutrients are in the food. The serving size information may also be helpful to individuals who are practicing portion control, as the serving size could be used as to indicate how much a patient should eat if he is trying to limit his caloric intake.

Because weight loss cannot be achieved without a caloric deficit, the clinician should show the patient where he can find the calorie information on the nutrition facts label. The calorie information is located below the lines for serving size and number of servings per container. The clinician should emphasize that the calories listed only pertain to one serving, so if the patient consumes multiple servings, he will need to multiply the calories by the number of servings he consumes.

Additional nutrient information is also available on the nutrition facts label. Grams of various types of fats and carbohydrates are listed, as are the grams of protein. Labels may also list percent daily values for the various macro- and micronutrients, and these percentages are based on a 2,000 kcal diet. Because most weight management patients will not need 2,000 cal, these percentages may not be as helpful as simply focusing on the calories and absolute amounts of various macro- and micronutrients.

Besides the nutrient and serving size information, another component of the nutrition facts label is the ingredients statement. This statement appears below the main portion of the nutrition facts panel. In this statement, the actual ingredients of the food or beverage are listed in decreasing order by weight. For example, a product whose ingredient statement includes tomatoes, distilled vinegar, and high fructose corn syrup will contain more tomatoes by weight than distilled vinegar or high fructose corn syrup.

In some weight management programs, patients may be encouraged to read these ingredients statements and eliminate any foods that have added sugar as one of the first three ingredients. Although this practice is not promoted in all clinics, it may help some patients with reducing empty calories from added sugar in their diets. Ingredients statements are also helpful for patients who must avoid certain foods or food items for allergy purposes. For example, a patient with a peanut allergy should read all the ingredients statements to ensure that the products they consume do not contain peanuts.

Planning and Preparing Meals

When meals are prepared by the patient, the patient will have control over what foods and ingredients are used, how much of these foods and ingredients are used, and how the foods are finally prepared. All of these factors have a major impact on the caloric content of a meal; therefore, it is advantageous for weight management patients limiting their caloric intake to prepare their own meals whenever possible.

Research has shown that home-prepared meals tend to be lower in calories than meals prepared away from the home (i.e., store-prepared and restaurant-prepared meals) (Guthrie, Lin, and Frazao 2002, 140–50), and individuals who consume more meals prepared at home consume fewer calories than those who frequently eat foods prepared away from the home (Poti and Popkin 2011, 1156–64).

Nevertheless, although it seems that this simple recommendation (i.e., prepare meals and eat at home more often) would be an easy strategy for weight loss, patients report a multitude of barriers to following this recommendation. To many patients, the process of planning and preparing meals can be a daunting one. This process takes a significant amount of time and energy on behalf of the patient, and for those with busy lives, planning and preparing meals every day may not be an option. However, the process of planning and preparing meals can be made easier if the patient and the clinician work together to devise an initial meal plan inclusive of simple and healthy recipes.

At the beginning of a weight management program, the clinician should ask the patient about his meal planning and food preparation skills. This will identify a baseline for the patient, and the clinician can help the patient to improve these skills throughout the program. If the patient has never formally planned or prepared meals, then the clinician should work with the patient to develop an initial meal plan that involves minimal food preparation. When developing the meal plan, the clinician will need to know what food preparation and cooking equipment the patient has; examples of these pieces of equipment are listed in Box 8.3. The clinician may also want to help the patient devise a grocery list in order to simplify the shopping process.

Box 8.3 Common food preparation and cooking equipment used by weight management patients

Food preparation equipment:

- Can opener
- Cutting board
- Knife set
- Grater
- Measuring cups
- Mixing bowls
- Peeler
- Pots and pans
- Potholder
- Teaspoons and tablespoons
- Utensils

Small appliances:

- Blender
- Food processor
- Griddle or countertop grill
- Hot plate
- Mixer
- Pressure cooker
- Rice cooker

Slow cooker
Thermometer
Toaster or toaster oven

Large appliances:

Dishwasher
Freezer
Microwave
Grill
Stove
Refrigerator
Oven

If the patient does have some experience with planning meals and preparing foods, the clinician should focus more on what types of foods the patient typically prepares and how those foods could be modified to be healthier. For example, if the patient states that he makes chicken and rice at least once a week, then the clinician should ask how the chicken is prepared and what ingredients he adds to the rice. If the patient states that he fries the chicken and boils the rice, the clinician should recommend changing the chicken to baked or grilled chicken because it is lower in calories than fried chicken.

Box 8.4 lists the various food preparation methods, which should be used by patients who are attempting to lose weight. The clinician should find out if the patient is familiar with these techniques and suggest that the patient utilize these methods over other methods, which could increase the caloric content of meals (e.g., frying and sautéing).

Box 8.4 Recommended food preparation methods for weight management patients

Dry heat methods:

Bake
Broil

(*Continued*)

(*Continued*)

Grill
Roast

Moist heat methods (using water or other no or low-calorie liquid):

Braise
Boil
Poach
Simmer
Steam
Stew

Meal Frequency

Patients who are trying to lose weight may be tempted to skip meals in order to save calories and further their caloric deficit. However, skipping meals can be detrimental to weight loss goals as it may intensify hunger and lead to overeating at meals. In order to keep a patient on track, the patient's meal plan should reflect multiple eating occasions throughout the day.

Individuals will typically schedule meals at habitual times or around other daily activities; however, these meal times may not always be conducive to weight management. When they are not, it is the clinician's responsibility to assist the patient with properly planning his mealtimes and help the patient develop a more normal schedule of eating.

Most patients should be advised to eat breakfast every morning soon after they awaken. Skipping breakfast has been associated with obesity (De la Hunty and Ashwell 2007, 118–28; Ma et al. 2003, 85–92; Szajewska and Ruszczyński 2010, 113–19), whereas regular breakfast consumption is a common trait among individuals who have lost weight and managed to keep the weight off (Wyatt et al. 2002, 78–82). Children, in particular, should be encouraged to consume breakfast (Berkey et al. 2003, 1258–66) not only because of the weight-related benefits but also because of breakfast consumption's association with cognitive function and academic performance (Rampersaud et al. 2005, 743–60).

The timing and spacing of other meals, besides breakfast, may also be helpful for patients who are trying to manage their weight. Eating four or more times per day has been linked to lower risk of obesity (Ma et al. 2003, 85–92) in adults, and consuming five or more meals has been linked to lower risk of obesity in children (Toschke et al. 2005, 1932–38). As such, it may behoove the clinician to devise a meal plan inclusive of at least three meals and one to two small snacks for patients who are seeking weight management. However, the overall caloric content must be analyzed in order keep the patient in a caloric deficit. Although the timing of meals may be disrupted during special events and holidays, clinicians should encourage patients to adhere to the meal plan as closely as possible to instill the habit of regular eating.

Clinicians may also want to encourage their patients to avoid eating late at night. Although calories are calories, regardless of the time of day ingested, patients may have a tendency to snack on less healthy items or to eat more mindlessly in the late evening. This is also something that clinicians should look for when evaluating patients' food records.

Meal Replacements

For some patients, consuming three meals per day is challenging, especially when each meal needs to be planned and prepared. To avoid this challenge and facilitate a more rapid weight loss, many patients may turn to meal replacements or substitutes. Meal replacements typically come in the form of snack-sized bars or liquid nutrition drinks, and are consumed in lieu of other foods as a meal. Because they are being consumed by themselves, these replacements are specially formulated to include a variety of vitamins and minerals and contain all of the three essential macronutrients.

Patients using these nutrition drinks or bars in lieu of meals should only do so while under medical supervision. In some cases, patients taking meal replacements may over restrict their caloric intake, and this can result in metabolic abnormalities or extreme hunger and bingeing. Clinicians should familiarize themselves with the popular brands of meal replacements available on the market and decide which replacement is most appropriate for the patient. For example, if a patient is following a carbohydrate-restricted diet, a low-carbohydrate, high-protein meal replacement supplement may be more desirable than a low-fat meal replacement.

The clinician determines how many times a meal replacement should be consumed each day. Some studies have demonstrated weight loss success with replacing only one or two meals per day (Ashley et al. 2001, 312S–20S; Heymsfield et al. 2003, 537–49; Noakes et al. 2004, 1894–99); however, the clinician may recommend replacing meals more often than this, particularly when a patient is first starting a program.

When meal replacements are used in a weight management program, the patient's diet should be carefully monitored for nutritional adequacy. Although meal replacements are specifically formulated to include multiple essential nutrients, it is often difficult for patients to meet all their nutritional requirements when consuming multiple replacements and very little food. In addition, most meal replacements lack the antioxidants and phytochemicals found in plant-based foods. As such, a variety of fresh fruits and nonstarchy vegetables may still be recommended when a patient is taking multiple replacements each day.

Typically, the concept of using meal replacements is not a difficult one to convey to patients; however, it is extremely important that patients know the exact brand of replacement they need to consume and when and how often they need to consume it. Patients may find it helpful to continue following a meal plan that outlines when they are to consume the replacements, such as the one seen in Box 8.5.

Box 8.5 Example of a 1,200 kcal meal plan including two meal replacements

Patient: John Doe
DOB: 1/3/52
Sex: Male
Age: 64 years
Breakfast @ 06:30:

11 oz meal replacement drink (~240 kcal)

Morning snack @ 10:00:

1 cup strawberries
5 oz Greek yogurt

Lunch @ 12:00:

11 oz meal replacement drink (~240 kcal)

Afternoon snack @ 15:00:

4 small stalks celery
1 tbsp almond butter

Dinner:

4 oz grilled steak, lean
1 cup cooked spinach
1 small (5 inches) sweet potato with 1 tbsp butter
16 oz water
Total calories: 1,199 kcal

Summary

The basic concepts reviewed in this chapter are crucial to the success of any weight management program. Although patients cannot be expected to know all aspects of nutrition and diet, they should have a general understanding of how their dietary intake impacts their weight status and what behaviors they need to perform in order to create a caloric deficit and lose weight.

References

Ashley, J.M., S.T. Jeor, S. Perumean-Chaney, J. Schrage, and V. Bovee. 2001. "Meal Replacements in Weight Intervention." *Obesity Research* 9, no. S11, pp. 312S–20S. doi:10.1038/oby.2001.136

Berkey, C.S., H.R.H. Rockett, M.W. Gillman, A.E. Field, and G.A. Colditz. 2003. "Longitudinal Study of Skipping Breakfast and Weight Change in Adolescents." *International Journal of Obesity* 27, no. 10, pp. 1258–66. doi:10.1038/sj.ijo.0802402

Camelon, K.M., K. Hådell, P.Ä.I.V.I.T. Jämsén, K.J. Ketonen, H.M. Kohtamäki, S. Mäkimatilla, M.L. Törmälä, R.H. Valve, and DAIS Project Group. 1998. "The Plate Model: A Visual Method of Teaching Meal Planning." *Journal of the American Dietetic Association* 98, no. 10, pp. 1155–58. doi:10.1016/S0002-8223(98)00267-3

De la Hunty, A., and M. Ashwell. 2007. "Are People Who Regularly Eat Breakfast Cereals Slimmer than Those Who Don't? A Systematic Review of the Evidence." *Nutrition Bulletin* 32, no. 2, pp. 118–28. doi:10.1111/j.1467-3010.2007.00638.x

Guthrie, J.F., B.H. Lin, and E. Frazao. 2002. "Role of Food Prepared Away from Home in the American Diet, 1977–78 Versus 1994–96: Changes and Consequences." *Journal of Nutrition Education and Behavior* 34, no. 3, pp. 140–50. doi:10.1016/s1499-4046(06)60083-3

Heymsfield, S.B., C.A.J. Van Mierlo, H.C.M. Van der Knaap, M. Heo, and H.I. Frier. 2003. "Weight Management Using a Meal Replacement Strategy: Meta and Pooling Analysis from Six Studies." *International Journal of Obesity* 27, no. 5, pp. 537–49. doi:10.1038/sj.ijo.0802258

Klara, R. 2004. "Table the Issue." *Restaurant Business* 103, no. 18, pp. 14–15.

Lin, B.H., and J.F. Guthrie. 2012. "Nutritional Quality of Food Prepared at Home and Away from Home, 1977–2008." U.S. Department of Agriculture Economic Research Service.

Ma, Y., E.R. Bertone, E.J. Stanek 3rd, G.W. Reed, J.R. Hebert, N.L. Cohen, P.A. Merriam, and I.S. Ockene. 2003. "Association Between Eating Patterns and Obesity in a Free-Living US Adult Population." *American Journal of Epidemiology* 158, no. 1, pp. 85–92. doi:10.1093/aje/kwg117

Neuhouser, M.L., A.R. Kristal, and R.E. Patterson. 1999. "Use of Food Nutrition Labels Is Associated with Lower Fat Intake." *Journal of the American Dietetic Association* 99, no. 1, pp. 45–53. doi:10.1016/s0002-8223(99)00013-9

Noakes, M., P.R. Foster, J.B. Keogh, and P.M. Clifton. 2004. "Meal Replacements Are as Effective as Structured Weight-Loss Diets for Treating Obesity in Adults with Features of Metabolic Syndrome." *The Journal of Nutrition* 134, no. 8, pp. 1894–99.

Poti, J.M., and B.M. Popkin. 2011. "Trends in Energy Intake Among US Children by Eating Location and Food Source, 1977–2006." *Journal of the American Dietetic Association* 111, no. 8, pp. 1156–64. doi:10.1016/j.jada.2011.05.007

Rampersaud, G.C., M.A. Pereira, B.L. Girard, J. Adams, and J.D. Metzl. 2005. "Breakfast Habits, Nutritional Status, Body Weight, and Academic Performance in Children and Adolescents." *Journal of the American Dietetic Association* 105, no. 5, pp. 743–60. doi:10.1016/j.jada.2005.02.007

Szajewska, H., and M. Ruszczyński. 2010. "Systematic Review Demonstrating that Breakfast Consumption Influences Body Weight Outcomes in Children and Adolescents in Europe." *Critical Reviews in Food Science and Nutrition* 50, no. 2, pp. 113–19. doi:10.1080/10408390903467514

Temple, J.L., K. Johnson, K. Recupero, and H. Suders. 2011. "Nutrition Labels Decrease Energy Intake in Adults Consuming Lunch in the Laboratory." *Journal of the American Dietetic Association* 111, no. 5, pp. S52–55. doi:10.1016/j.jada.2011.03.010

Toschke, A.M., H. Küchenhoff, B. Koletzko, and R. Kries. 2005. "Meal Frequency and Childhood Obesity." *Obesity Research* 13, no. 11, pp. 1932–38. doi:10.1038/oby.2005.238

Wyatt, H.R., G.K. Grunwald, C.L. Mosca, M.L. Klem, R.R. Wing, and J.O. Hill. 2002. "Long-Term Weight Loss and Breakfast in Subjects in the National Weight Control Registry." *Obesity Research* 10, no. 2, pp. 78–82. doi:10.1038/oby.2002.13

CHAPTER 9

Weight Loss Intervention: Behavior Modification

Dietary intake is a deeply engrained and extremely complex human behavior. As such, modifying this behavior can be challenging, and it may take several months (or even years) to establish new dietary habits. In this chapter, strategies for modifying dietary behaviors will be explored and examples for using these strategies will be discussed.

Self-Monitoring

There is strong evidence supporting the role of self-monitoring in modifying and improving dietary behaviors among adult (Academy of Nutrition and Dietetics 2014) and pediatric (Academy of Nutrition and Dietetics 2007, 11) patients who are trying to lose weight. Self-monitoring activities include having a patient document everything he eats and drinks during the day in a paper or electronic logbook. Self-monitoring activities can also include documenting where he consumes his meals, what time he consumes his meals, and how he is feeling at the time of consumption.

Self-monitoring can then be used as a tool for reflection. For example, if a patient logs everything he eats for a week, then he and the clinician can review the logbook at their visit and identify trends. The patient may notice that he tends to eat empty calorie foods in the evening when he is tired and is watching television, or he may notice that he eats fast food more often than he originally thought.

Self-monitoring logs can be analyzed for nutrient and food content by the Registered Dietitian Nutritionist (RDN). Findings from this kind of analysis should be shared with the patient and used to modify the meal plan. For example, if the RDN analyzes a patient's weekly intake record and finds that the patient only consumes an average of 15 g fiber per day, then the RDN should work with the patient to modify the meal plan to incorporate more high fiber foods.

Motivational Interviewing

When attempting to modify a patient's dietary behavior, motivation interviewing (MI) is another strategy that can be used. Although MI was originally founded as a technique to help alcoholics recover from problematic drinking (Miller 1983, 147–72; Miller and Rollnick 1991), over the years, it has also been associated with eliciting dietary change among both adult (Elder, Ayala, and Harris 1999, 275–84) and pediatric (Resnicow, Davis, and Rollnick 2006, 2024–33) patients. MI is intended for individuals who may be reluctant to change their dietary patterns or who may be ambivalent to change. The goal of MI is to help the patient find his own intrinsic motivation to make the desired change.

The MI process is led by a clinician who asks a series of nonjudgmental, open-ended questions. These questions prompt the patient to fully explore his motivations to perform (or in some cases, not perform) a certain dietary behavior. By asking these questions, the patient is encouraged to discuss his feelings about a certain behavior and what the rationales for those feelings are. Throughout the interview, the clinician affirms what the patient says, in order to show empathy and encouragement. This will also help the patient be more truthful and honest in his answers.

Once the patient answers an open-ended question, the clinician reflects on what he hears the patient saying and summarizes what he hears. This allows the patient to clarify anything that may have been misconstrued, and it also allows the patient to hear his own words from another source. Many times, hearing his own words paraphrased by another individual will help a patient identify inconsistencies in his own logic or will highlight specific details that the patient may not have felt were important.

During the interview, a clinician gives the patient the opportunity to identify pros and cons of the behavior. Allowing the patient to discuss these benefits and drawbacks gives the patient an opportunity to weight these characteristics and make a fully informed decision. This strategy, known as decisional balance, is a key part of MI.

Throughout the MI process, the clinician should always keep a kind, empathetic tone and should avoid any judgmental terms or confrontational language. The clinician should support the patient's self-efficacy to make behavior change by focusing on the positive aspects of the behavior while acknowledging that change is difficult for most people. Examples of questions and statements used during MI are seen in Box 9.1.

Box 9.1 ***Example questions and statements for motivational interviewing***

Open-ended questions: Use questions like these to start the conversation.

- Tell me how you feel about your current weight or health status.
- How would you describe your current diet?
- Rate your diet on a scale of 1–5, with 5 being a healthy diet and 1 being an unhealthy diet. Why did you rate your diet as a [X]?
- What's happened with your diet since our last visit?
- Who are the most important people in your life? How do they impact your food intake?

Decisional balance questions: Ask these questions to help the patient explore the pros and cons of the desired behavior.

- What do you like about eating fast food? What do you dislike about it?
- What makes eating healthy easy? What makes it difficult?
- What are some of the good things about …? On the opposite side, what are some of the bad things about …?
- What do you enjoy about exercising? What do you dislike about exercising?

Reflection statements: Once a patient has answered a question, use this kind of statements to restate what he has just told you.

- What I hear you telling me is …
- Based on what you've told me, it sounds like …
- Let me recap what I've heard you say …

(*Continued*)

(*Continued*)

- It sounds to me like …
- I am sensing that you …

Affirmation statements: Use these statements to acknowledge a patient's successes.

- You have clearly demonstrated a commitment to the meal plan by …
- Despite how busy your life is, it's clear that you're committed to changing your lifestyle because you …
- You showed a lot of dedication this past week by …

Structured Meal Plans

Although self-monitoring can help patients to track what they consume, patients may also need specific guidance on what to consume in order to create a caloric deficit and lose weight. As such, structured meal plans may be recommended. These plans will include the exact types and quantities of food a patient should plan to consume each day, and they should be labeled with the day and time when patients should consume the items.

A structured meal plan can be especially helpful when patients are first starting a weight management program because planning meals and picking out healthier foods can be overwhelming to patients who have little training in nutrition. Having a structured meal plan to follow can alleviate some of this stress and anxiety because the patient will not have to decide what or how much to eat; instead, he will simply follow the plan.

Another added benefit of the structured meal plan is that it guides patients when they are in the grocery store. These plans indicate exactly what the patient needs to buy and may keep some patients from purchasing additional foods and beverages that contribute to overeating. Following a structured meal plan at the grocery store can also help contain the costs of food because patients will only buy what is on the plan.

The degree to which meal plans are structured can vary. In general, meal plans need to be the most structured at the beginning of the weight management program when a patient is first establishing new dietary habits. Later in the program, the patient may require less structure as he has established better habits and is more attuned to internal hunger cues and more able to select lower calorie foods on his own.

As much as possible, flexibility should be incorporated into structured meal plans. This will assist with feasibility of implementation and can increase the likelihood that a patient will adhere to the diet. For example, if a structured meal plan has a small banana with breakfast, then the clinician could also give the patient the option of having a different fruit with approximately the same number of calories and a similar nutritional value (e.g., a medium apple or pear instead of the banana). Box 9.2 shows a structured meal plan with appropriate options so as not to bore the patient.

Box 9.2 ***Example of structured meal plan with options for breakfast***

Breakfast—consume @ 07:00 on weekdays and 08:00 on weekend days

- 1 cup cooked oatmeal (Option A: 1–1/2 cup dry oat cereal, Option B: 2 slices whole wheat toast)
- 3/4 cup blueberries (Option A: 1/2 medium banana, Option B: 1 small orange)
- 1 cup 1% milk (Option A: 5 oz light Greek yogurt, Option B: 6 oz light yogurt)
- 2 tsp butter (Option A: 12 almonds, 2 tbsp. flax seeds)

Goal Setting

As discussed in Chapter 6, it is important to set goals such as target weights when starting a weight management program. However, the number on the scale should never be the only goal of a weight management program. Instead, goals should also include new, healthier behaviors related to dietary intake and physical activity.

The act of setting behaviorally focused goals should be a collaborative one that involves both the clinician and the patient. Although the clinician may know what the patient needs to do in order to lose weight, the patient may not be ready or willing to perform this behavior. As such, it is important for the clinician and the patient to set goals that are SMART and will move the patient in the right direction.

More information on goal setting and example goals can be found in Chapter 6.

Problem-Solving

For most individuals, modifying their dietary behaviors poses a number of challenges. There are a myriad of barriers that can prevent the selection and consumption of healthy foods, and these barriers or problems may seem overwhelming to someone who is just starting a weight management program.

It is the clinician's responsibility to help the patient problem-solve the barriers to and challenges associated with making healthy food selections. The clinician must recognize that each patient will present with his own unique challenges, and what may be a difficult situation or problem for one patient may not necessarily be the case with all patients.

When conducting a problem-solving session with a patient, the clinician can use MI to elicit specific information about the problem. Together with the patient, the clinician should devise a plan to conquer the problem, and steps in this plan will be part of the behavioral goals for the patient. At future encounters, the clinician should follow-up with the patient to gauge the effectiveness of the problem-solving strategies.

One of the common problems patients may have is around dining at restaurants. For example, a patient may say that he has to eat at a full-service restaurant at least twice a week with his work clients. When dining out, the patient may tend to overindulge and consume excess calories. Given this situation, the clinician should probe the patient about these experiences and help the patient to problem solve the issues. Once a plan is developed, the clinician should document the plan, give a copy of the plan to the patient, then plan to discuss how well the patient implemented the plan at their follow-up encounter. An example of a problem-solving plan for this situation can be seen in Box 9.3.

Box 9.3 An example of a problem-solving plan for eating out at restaurants with work clients

Patient: John Doe
DOB: 1/3/52
Sex: Male
Age: 64 years
Problem:

Difficulty with making healthy food selections when dining out at restaurants with work clients

Solution:

Before arriving at the restaurant:

- Prior to going to the restaurant, look up the restaurant online. Find the nutrition information. Find a dish with less than 500 kcal per meal, and plan to order this dish.
- If nutrition information is not available, find simple protein-based dish (e.g., grilled salmon, baked chicken) without sauce, and plan to order it with steamed vegetables.

While at the restaurant:

- Order seltzer water instead of an alcoholic beverage at happy hour.
- Order a side salad with balsamic vinegar for appetizer. If desired, could substitute with a small, broth-based vegetable soup.
- Instead of desert, order a decaffeinated coffee with skim milk.

After returning home:

- Document everything consumed in food log.

Cognitive Restructuring

Cognitive restructuring is an advanced psychotherapy technique that can be used to change the thinking and thought processes of those patients seeking weight management guidance. While traditionally used among patients seeking therapy for social anxiety, cognitive restructuring is a successful strategy for reframing negative thoughts and feelings toward oneself (Hope et al. 2010, 1–12).

The first step of cognitive restructuring is identifying the patient's thoughts that are detrimental to the treatment goal. In weight management patients, these negative thoughts are usually related to food and dieting, but they will be specific to the patient. For example, a patient may exhibit a detrimental, all-or-nothing mentality when he says, "I stepped on the scale and saw my weight was up 2 lb, so I was like, forget it! And I just ate a huge cheeseburger with French fries for dinner." The clinician should readily identify any dysfunctional thinking that could lead to program failure and be willing to discuss it with the patient.

The next step of cognitive restructuring is fleshing out the thought processes associated with the dysfunctional thought. In this step, the clinician probes the patient to better understand how the thoughts influenced the behavior, but more importantly, the clinician tries to get the patient to see how irrational the thought is or how disconnected and inappropriate the behavior is. In the example above, the clinician might ask the patient why he felt it was appropriate to eat something that was not on his meal plan. This kind of question might prompt the patient to say he felt like a failure because his weight had not decreased. Then the clinician could ask the patient to explain why his weight may not have decreased, and the patient could potentially explain it by saying he was wearing heavier clothes or had drank more water that day. These realizations may be something the patient had not previously considered.

Now that the clinician has helped the patient to think more rationally, the final step of cognitive restructuring is prevention of future irrational thinking. In this step, clinicians need to help patients with developing coping mechanisms for identifying and diffusing future dysfunctional thoughts in an effort to prevent setbacks and relapses.

Overall, the process of cognitive restructuring can be time and resource intensive, and it innately requires a good clinician–patient relationship; however, its return on investment is high and the strategy is well worthwhile.

Contingency Management

Contingency management is a strategy that has been successfully used in substance abuse and mental health treatment (Stitzer and Petry 2006,

411–34), but it can also be useful in weight management programs. In contingency management, a patient is incentivized to perform a specific behavior because in doing so, he will receive some kind of reward, often in the form of a voucher that can be redeemed for some material item.

In weight management programs, contingency management is often used among pediatric patients. For example, a clinician may incentivize a young patient to eat five different fruits and vegetables each day by telling him that he will receive a sticker on each day which he does so. For adult patients, contingency management is still appropriate, and the reward should be something the adult values and something he can commit to doing for himself if he achieves the goal. For example, a female patient may want to get a manicure if she can achieve the goal of exercising 30 minutes each day for 2 weeks. The reward does not have to be funded by the clinician; however, the clinician should assist the patient in identifying the reward so he can hold the patient accountable in claiming the reward once the patient achieves it.

When devising an appropriate reward for contingency management, the clinician should find out what would appeal most to the patient. After all, the reward is part of what will motivate the patient to perform the behavior and meet the behavioral goal. The reward should be mutually agreed upon by the patient and the clinician, and it should be feasible and reasonable. Food-based incentives should never be used as part of contingency management, as this would undermine the program's goals and reinforce an inappropriate use of food. Examples of appropriate rewards are seen in Box 9.4.

Box 9.4 Examples of rewards or incentives for a weight management program

Pediatric patients:

- Stickers
- Pencils or pens
- Crayons and coloring books
- Temporary tattoos
- Tickets to local museum

(*Continued*)

(*Continued*)

- Extra play time at the park
- Movie matinee (be careful about purchasing food at the movie theater)
- Special board game night

Female adult patients:

- Manicure or pedicure
- Massage
- New book or magazine
- Mom's night off (ensure family commits to giving mom a night off from her normal duties)

Male adult patients:

- Sporting event (be mindful to discuss the food environments of sports venues as they may not be conducive to healthy eating)
- New book or magazine
- New exercise or fitness equipment
- Special hobby-related class
- Dad's night off (ensure family commits to giving mom a night off from her normal duties)

Relapse Prevention

As discussed in the section on cognitive restructuring, preventing negative thoughts and feelings is key to the success of a weight management program. In addition, preventing the patient from reverting to old bad habits is also imperative. During each encounter, clinicians should discuss the steps necessary to prevent behavior relapses and ensure that the patient has the appropriate skills to cope with potential relapses. This is especially important when patients will not be seen by the clinician for several weeks or months.

Clinicians can broach the subject of relapse prevention by creating hypothetical situations. For example, the clinician may ask the patient, "What would you do if you stepped on the scale and saw your weight was higher than last week?" or "How would you get back on track if you splurged at dinner one night?" These questions force the patient to articulate what behaviors he would perform, making it somewhat more likely he will perform those behaviors in the future.

Another strategy for preventing relapses in between visits is to ensure that the patient has the appropriate social support to get him back on track. The clinician may ask the patient to identify a friend or family member who could help hold him accountable during times when the patient is struggling to continue the proper behaviors or stick to new, healthier habits. This support individual should be reliable and should be someone the patient is comfortable with contacting and discussing sensitive information.

Stress Management

Stress can affect individuals in a number of ways; some people will eat less when they are stressed, and others will eat more. Stress causes a surge in hormones, which can also alter the way a person behaves and conducts himself. Because stress can have a negative impact on human physiology and behavior, it is important that clinicians help their patients manage stress in a constructive manner that does not hinder weight management progress.

Patients who frequently experience high-stress situations should be encouraged to document their stress levels and feelings on their food log. This will allow the clinician to determine how a patient reacts to stress and how that reaction may be impacting weight management success. For example, Box 9.5 shows a food log written by a patient who reports a lot of stress at work. In this example, the clinician may notice that the patient appears to get stressed at work, and when he does, his dietary behavior changes. This would then prompt the clinician to discuss effective stress management techniques with the patient and encourage the patient to utilize these techniques in situations where stress will occur.

Box 9.5 Example of food log with accompanying stress and feelings documentation

Name: John Doe

Date of food log entry: Monday, January 11, 2016

Meal, time, and location	Food and amount	Stress level (1 = no stress, 5 = high stress) and feelings
Breakfast 08:00 Home, at kitchen table	8 oz coffee with 2 tsp sugar 1 small apple	2, Running late, feeling frantic
Snack 10:30 Work, at desk	5 oz Greek yogurt, light	1, Not stressed
Snack 11:15 Work, at desk	5 chocolate kisses 12 oz Diet Coke	4, After stressful meeting, upset about new work assignment
Lunch 14:00 Car	1 cheeseburger with ketchup, lettuce, tomato, mayo 1 medium French fries 16 oz Diet Coke	5, Late lunch, very hungry, stressed because I missed my healthy lunch
Snack 16:30 Work, at desk	1 medium chocolate bar from vending machine	3, Upset about colleague, mad that I ate fast food at lunch

When possible, it is ideal to eliminate the sources of stress which result in an undesirable behavior. For example, if a patient knows that eating while in the office and surrounded by colleagues will induce stress, the patient should be encouraged to eat outside of this environment. Similarly, if a patient acknowledges that certain people will induce stress by encouraging him to eat foods that are not conducive to weight loss, the patient should be encouraged to limit food consumption while around these people.

It is important to recognize, however, that not all stresses can be eliminated, and when this is the case, mechanisms for positively coping with the stressor should be explored and implemented. The clinician and patient should work together to devise plans on how to cope with stressful environments and people. Positive coping mechanisms may include exercising or taking a walk, listening to relaxing music, meditating or praying, or writing in a journal. When possible, the patient should document using these positive coping mechanisms so the clinician can see that he is using these strategies successfully.

Environmental Considerations

In order to modify behaviors, patients may also need to modify the environment in which they eat. The people in that environment and the location of that environment can have a significant impact on food choices and calorie consumption. As such, the clinician should ensure these environments are discussed throughout the weight management program.

People

For the majority of people, mealtime is a social occasion that involves close companions, family members, and friends. However, the presence of these companions significantly influences food and caloric intake. Research has shown that when adults are with a companion, they may consume more food over a longer period of time than when they are eating alone (De Castro 1994, 445–55) or with strangers (Koh and Pliner 2009, 595–602). When eating with a partner, adults also tend to mimic their companion and consume their food at the same time as their companion (Hermans et al. 2012, e31027), potentially ignoring internal hunger and satiety cues.

In adolescents and children, eating with the family may have positive nutritional benefits. For example, one study demonstrated that adolescents who ate with their family had better intakes of fruits and vegetables and lower intakes of soft drinks (Neumark-Sztainer et al. 2003, 317–22). Other studies have shown that children who engage in family meals are less likely to be overweight (Gable, Chang, and Krull 2007, 53–61) and exhibit disordered eating patterns (Hammons and Fiese 2011, e1565–74). It should be noted, however, that family meals may not be as beneficial if the parents are pressuring their children to eat specific foods, as this pressuring has been linked to low fruit and vegetable intake (Galloway et al. 2005, 541–48) and overeating (Fisher and Birch 2002, 226–31).

Because of the social nature of eating, it is important for weight management patients to consider with whom they consume meals and how these companions may potentially impact their intake. Along with the types and amounts of food consumed, the names and relationships of people at meals can be recorded in a patient's food diary, and the clinician can review this information at the same time he reviews the other information in the diary. The clinician should identify any person-specific trends in consumption and discuss this with the patient, especially when the trend is not conducive to weight management.

Location

Where a patient consumes his meals is often tied to who he is with and what he is doing at mealtime. Where he consumes his food can also be tied to the types of foods he consumes and their corresponding nutritional value.

Individuals frequently eat at the same location where the food is procured (i.e., a restaurant, fast food establishment, home), thus making the meal contents dependent of the foods that are available at that location. For example, if a patient eats in a restaurant, he will only be able to consume the food that is available at that restaurant. This concept, known as food availability, is known to greatly influence dietary intake and diet quality (Franco et al. 2009, 897–904) simply because patients can only eat what is available to them. If healthy foods are not available, then the patient will have to consume less healthy foods that may not be conducive to weight management.

Most patients will report eating out at restaurants and fast food establishments at least once per week, and this can become problematic if the patient makes high-calorie choices when dining at these locations. Clinicians should encouraged patients to seek out the nutrition information for menu items before eating out or to ask for this information when at the establishment. Having this information will help them make an informed choice about what they consume and may help them stay within their caloric allotment for the meal. Patients should also be encouraged to limit their portion sizes when dining out, and to ensure that they fill up on lower calorie, vegetable-based items such as salads, vegetable soups, and steamed vegetables.

Depending on their age, most patients will also report eating while at work or at school. Food availability at these locations can vary widely, thus making it important for the patient to consider what foods are available in these locations and how conducive these foods are to his weight management goals. Although much emphasis has been placed on improving healthy food availability in workplaces (Quintiliani, Sattelmair, and Sorensen 2007), healthy foods are still not available in many locations. As such, clinicians should encourage their patients to bring healthy foods with them to consume while at work.

Food availability at schools in the United States has been improving over the past few years. Starting in 2012, the U.S. Department of Agriculture instituted new nutritional guidelines that set standards on the types and amounts of foods that could be sold in primary and secondary schools that participate in the federally funded child nutrition programs (i.e., National School Lunch and School Breakfast Programs) (U.S. Department of Agriculture, Food and Nutrition Service 2012, 2013). These new guidelines improved the nutritional content of foods available during school hours and set limits on the number of calories reimbursable meals could contain. However, not all children eat these meals; thus clinicians should be mindful of the types and amounts of foods pediatric patients consume while at school. If a patient does eat from the school cafeteria, the clinician may want to review the foods being offered in the cafeteria and verify that the patient's selections are appropriate and conducive to weight management. If the patient does not eat from the school cafeteria, the clinician should assist the patient in developing a plan for what kinds of and how much food the patient should bring to school.

When patients consume meals at home or at work, they may be tempted to consume these meals while watching television. When possible, this should be discouraged. Individuals who eat while watching television are prone to eat more food than when not watching television (Braude and Stevenson 2014, 9–16; Ogden et al. 2013, 119–26), and this can potentially lead to overconsumption of calories. Patients should be encouraged to be mindful and attentive to their food consumption when eating, and distractions such as the television should be minimized.

Summary

In order to properly engage patients and ensure their behaviors are conducive to good health and weight loss, behavior modification strategies should be used. Although not all strategies may be effective for all patients, the clinician should attempt to implement them in order to maximize program effectiveness and prevent barriers from impeding progress.

References

Academy of Nutrition and Dietetics. 2007. "Pediatric Weight Management: Executive Summary of Recommendations." www.andeal.org/topic.cfm?menu=5296&cat=3013 (accessed June, 2015).

Academy of Nutrition and Dietetics. 2014. "Adult Weight Management: Executive Summary of Recommendations." www.andeal.org/topic.cfm?menu=5276&cat=4690 (accessed July 2, 2015).

Braude, L., and R.J. Stevenson. 2014. "Watching Television while Eating Increases Energy Intake. Examining the Mechanisms in Female Participants." *Appetite* 76, pp. 9–16. doi:10.1016/j.appet.2014.01.005

De Castro, J.M. 1994. "Family and Friends Produce Greater Social Facilitation of Food Intake than Other Companions." *Physiology and Behavior* 56, no. 3, pp. 445–55. doi:10.1016/0031-9384(94)90286-0

Elder, J.P., G.X. Ayala, and S. Harris. 1999. "Theories and Intervention Approaches to Health-Behavior Change in Primary Care." *American Journal of Preventive Medicine* 17, no. 4, pp. 275–84. doi:10.1016/s0749-3797(99)00094-x

Fisher, J.O., and L.L. Birch. 2002. "Eating in the Absence of Hunger and Overweight in Girls from 5 to 7 y of Age." *The American Journal of Clinical Nutrition* 76, no. 1, pp. 226–31.

Franco, M., A.V. Diez-Roux, J.A. Nettleton, M. Lazo, F. Brancati, B. Caballero, T. Glass, and L.V. Moore. 2009. "Availability of Healthy Foods and Dietary Patterns: The Multi-Ethnic Study of Atherosclerosis." *The American Journal of Clinical Nutrition* 89, no. 3, pp. 897–904. doi:10.3945/ajcn.2008.26434

Gable, S., Y. Chang, and J.L. Krull. 2007. "Television Watching and Frequency of Family Meals Are Predictive of Overweight Onset and Persistence in a National Sample of School-Aged Children." *Journal of the American Dietetic Association* 107, no. 1, pp. 53–61. doi:10.1016/j.jada.2006.10.010

Galloway, A.T., L. Fiorito, Y. Lee, and L.L. Birch. 2005. "Parental Pressure, Dietary Patterns, and Weight Status Among Girls Who Are 'Picky Eaters'." *Journal of the American Dietetic Association* 105, no. 4, pp. 541–48. doi:10.1016/j.jada.2005.01.029

Hammons, A.J., and B.H. Fiese. 2011. "Is Frequency of Shared Family Meals Related to the Nutritional Health of Children and Adolescents?" *Pediatrics* 127, no. 6, pp. e1565–74. doi:10.1542/peds.2010-1440

Hermans, R.C., A. Lichtwarck-Aschoff, K.E. Bevelander, C.P. Herman, J.K. Larsen, and R.C. Engels. 2012. "Mimicry of Food Intake: The Dynamic Interplay Between Eating Companions." *PloS One* 7, no. 2: e31027. doi:10.1371/journal.pone.0031027

Hope, D.A., J.A. Burns, S.A. Hayes, J.D. Herbert, and M.D. Warner. 2010. "Automatic Thoughts and Cognitive Restructuring in Cognitive Behavioral Group Therapy for Social Anxiety Disorder." *Cognitive Therapy and Research* 34, no. 1, pp. 1–12. doi:10.1007/s10608-007-9147-9

Koh, J., and P. Pliner. 2009. "The Effects of Degree of Acquaintance, Plate Size, and Sharing on Food Intake." *Appetite* 52, no. 3, pp. 595–602. doi:10.1016/j.appet.2009.02.004

Miller, W.R. 1983. "Motivational Interviewing with Problem Drinkers." *Behavioural Psychotherapy* 11, no. 2, pp. 147–72. doi:10.1017/s0141347300006583

Bennett, G. 1992. *Miller, W.R. and Rollnick, S. (1991) Motivational interviewing: Preparing people to change addictive behavior.* New York: Guilford Press. doi:10.1002/casp.2450020410

Neumark-Sztainer, D., P.J. Hannan, M. Story, J. Croll, and C. Perry. 2003. "Family Meal Patterns: Associations with Sociodemographic Characteristics and Improved Dietary Intake Among Adolescents." *Journal of the American Dietetic Association* 103, no. 3, pp. 317–22. doi:10.1053/jada.2003.50048

Ogden, J., N. Coop, C. Cousins, R. Crump, L. Field, S. Hughes, and N. Woodger. 2013. "Distraction, the Desire to Eat and Food Intake. Towards an Expanded Model of Mindless Eating." *Appetite* 62, pp. 119–26. doi:10.1016/j.appet.2012.11.023

Quintiliani, L., J. Sattelmair, and G. Sorensen. 2007. *Documento Técnico Preparado Para El Evento Conjunto OMS/Foro Económico Mundial Sobre La Prevención De Las Enfermedades no Transmisibles En El Lugar De Trabajo* [The Workplace as a Setting for Interventions to Improve Diet and Promote Physical Activity]. Ginebra: Organización Mundial De La Salud.

Resnicow, K., R. Davis, and S. Rollnick. 2006. "Motivational Interviewing for Pediatric Obesity: Conceptual Issues and Evidence Review." *Journal of the American Dietetic Association* 106, no. 12, pp. 2024–33. doi:10.1016/j.jada.2006.09.015

Stitzer, M., and N. Petry. 2006. "Contingency Management for Treatment of Substance Abuse." *Annual Review of Clinical Psychology* 2, pp. 411–34. doi:10.1146/annurev.clinpsy.2.022305.095219

U.S. Department of Agriculture, Food and Nutrition Service. 2012. "CFR Parts 210 and 220, Nutrition Standards in the National School Lunch and School Breakfast Programs; Final Rule." *Federal Register* 77, no. 17.

U.S. Department of Agriculture, Food and Nutrition Service. 2013. "7 CFR Parts 210 and 220, National School Lunch Program and School Breakfast Program: Nutrition Standards for All Foods Sold in School as Required by the Healthy, Hunger-Free Kids Act of 2010; Interim Final Rule." *Federal Register* 78, no. 125.

CHAPTER 10

Weight Loss Intervention: Medications

Individuals who are unable to lose weight through dietary modifications and physical activity may add prescription medications to their weight loss plan. Although the majority of these medications must be prescribed by authorized providers, they can further assist in some aspects of appetite and weight control; however, side effects and the duration of treatment must be carefully considered prior to initiating pharmacotherapy. This chapter will discuss the various types of medications that can assist with weight loss, how they achieve weight loss, and their potential side effects. (Please note that the medications discussed in this chapter should only be prescribed by physicians or clinicians with the appropriate order-writing privileges. This chapter is intended to serve as an overview of popular weight loss medications; however, it is not a substitute for the full prescribing information that is available through the manufacturer.)

Phentermine

Phentermine is the active ingredient in several well-known weight loss drugs, including Adipex-P® (Teva Pharmaceuticals, Mexico, MO) (Teva Pharmaceuticals USA 2014) and Qsymia® (VIVUS, Inc.) (VIVUS, Inc. 2015) (Qsymia will be discussed later in this chapter). In overweight and obese adults, phentermine-containing prescription drugs act by decreasing appetite and inducing weight loss when used in conjunction with a reduced calorie diet and exercise regimen (National Institutes of Health, National Library of Medicine 2015).

Phentermine drugs are available as a regular tablet that can be taken up to three times per day, or as an extended release capsule, which must only be taken once daily (National Institutes of Health, National

Library of Medicine 2015). Given that phentermine is chemically and pharmacologically similar to amphetamine, the medication is considered habit-forming, and as result, many phentermine-containing medications (e.g., Adipex-P) should only be taken for a maximum of 6 weeks.

The phentermine-containing medication Adipex-P is contraindicated in patients under 18 years, women who are pregnant and breastfeeding, and patients with a history of cardiovascular disease, glaucoma, hyperthyroidism, and drug abuse (Teva Pharmaceuticals USA 2014). Patients who have recently taken monoamine oxidase inhibitors (MAOIs) and patients in agitated states should avoid taking this medication. Before prescribing Adipex-P, clinicians should query patients about other drugs and supplements they are taking and gauge any potential drug–drug interactions.

Side effects of phentermine-containing medications include pulmonary hypertension, heart palpitations, elevated heart rate and blood pressure, and ischemic events. The drug may also cause patients to become dizzy and euphoric, both of which may impair a patient's ability to drive. In addition, nutrition-related side effects include, but are not limited to:

- Dry mouth
- Diarrhea
- Constipation
- Dysgeusia

Lorcaserin

Lorcaserin, the active ingredient in Belviq® (Eisai Inc./Arena Pharmaceuticals) (Arena Pharmaceuticals GmbH 2014), is a weight loss ingredient that was approved for use by the Food and Drug Administration (FDA) in 2012 (U.S. Department of Health and Human Services, Food and Drug Administration 2012a). Belviq, which is intended for long-term use in conjunction with diet and physical activity (Smith et al. 2010, 245–56), acts as a selective serotonin 2C receptor agonist and binds to the hypothalamus in order to reduce hunger.

Lorcaserin-containing medications (i.e., Belviq) are recommended as an adjunct therapy in adults with a body mass index (BMI) of at least 30 kg/m^2 or adults with a BMI of at least 27 kg/m^2 who also have one related comorbidity (e.g., high blood pressure, Type 2 diabetes mellitus (T2DM), elevated cholesterol) (U.S. Department of Health and Human Services, Food and Drug Administration 2012a). The recommended dosage is 10 mg by mouth, twice per day, and the medication can be taken with or without food.

Patients who are taking a lorcaserin-containing drug in conjunction with a reduced calorie diet and increased physical activity should experience a weight loss of 5 percent within 12 weeks (U.S. Department of Health and Human Services, Food and Drug Administration 2012a). If this weight loss does not occur by the end of 12 weeks, then the pharmacotherapy should be discontinued.

Lorcaserin-containing medications are only approved for adults and should not be used with children or adolescents under 18 years. The medication is contraindicated in women who are pregnant, and there are no current recommendations for using this medication while breastfeeding (National Institutes of Health, National Library of Medicine 2013). Lorcaserin drugs should not be used in patients with moderate or severe renal failure, and extreme caution should be used when prescribing the medication to those with severe hepatic impairment.

Nutrition-related side effects of lorcaserin-containing medications include, but are not limited to (Arena Pharmaceuticals GmbH 2015):

- Hypoglycemia
- Fatigue
- Nausea
- Dry mouth

Orlistat

Orlistat is an active ingredient in medications that promote weight loss by reducing the amount of dietary fat absorbed along the gastrointestinal tract. An orlistat-containing medication works as a lipase inhibitor, meaning that it inhibits the action of the lipase enzyme (Guerciolini 1997, S12–23). In particular, this medication selectively inhibits gastric and pancreatic lipases, which results in an incomplete breakdown of dietary fat. Because dietary fat is not fully digested, it cannot be absorbed and is, therefore, excreted from the body.

Orlistat-based medications is available in both prescription form, Xenical® (Genentech, Inc., Roche Group) (Genentech Inc., A member of the Roche Group 2012), and nonprescription form, Alli® (GlaxoSmithKline plc.) (GlaxoSmithKline 2013). The prescription form of the medication is available in a 120 mg dose, whereas the over-the-counter version is available in a 60 mg dose. The prescription form of orlistat has not been investigated in children under 12 years (Genentech Inc., A member of the Roche Group 2013), and the over-the-counter form of the drug is only recommended for adults ages 18 years and older (GlaxoSmithKline 2013).

Orlistat-containing medications can be taken multiple times each day, and it should be taken up to 1 hour before consuming a fat-containing meal in order to effectively inhibit the absorption of fat from the meal. When taking this medication, patients should follow a fat- and calorie-restricted diet along with an exercise regimen, and they should also limit the amount of total fat in a meal to no more than 15 g (GlaxoSmithKline 2013).

Orlistat-containing medications are is contraindicated in patients with chronic gastrointestinal malabsorption and in those with cholestasis (Genentech Inc., A member of the Roche Group 2013). Patients who are breastfeeding should not take Orlistat, and clinicians should exercise caution when prescribing it to breastfeeding mothers. Orlistat is also known to interact with numerous medications, including some anticoagulants and antiepileptic drugs.

Because of its mechanism of action, orlistat may inhibit the absorption of fat-soluble vitamins. As a result, the manufacturers recommend that patients taking orlistat also take a multivitamin supplement that contains the fat-soluble vitamins.

In 2010, the U.S. FDA issued a post-market drug safety communication on orlistat (U.S. Department of Health and Human Services, Food and Drug Administration 2010). Essentially, there had been a small number of reported cases of severe liver injury associated with taking orlistat, and as a result, FDA issued a statement requiring that manufacturers include information on severe liver injury on the drug's label. Although this side effect is rare, it should be taken into consideration along with the other nutrition-related side effects, which include but are not limited to (Genentech Inc., A member of the Roche Group 2013):

- Fatty and oily stools
- Flatus with discharge
- Increased stooling
- Fecal incontinence

Liraglutide

Liraglutide, the active ingredient in Saxenda® (Novo Nordisk) (Novo Nordisk A/S 2015a), is a prescription-only injectable medication, which received approval as a weight loss drug by FDA in 2014. Liraglutide is a glucagon-like peptide-1 (GLP-1) receptor agonist, which increases feelings of fullness and slows gastric emptying. As such, patients taking this medication may eat less and experience weight loss.

Liraglutide is also the active ingredient in Victoza® (Novo Nordisk) (Novo Nordisk A/S 2015b), a medication approved for use in patients with T2DM; however, the dose for Saxenda is less than the dose for treating diabetes (1.8 mg for Saxenda versus 3 mg for Victoza) (U.S. Department of Health and Human Services, Food and Drug Administration 2014). Saxenda should not be prescribed in conjunction with other liraglutide-containing medications or with insulin (Novo Nordisk A/S 2014).

When being prescribed for weight loss, liraglutide-containing medications should only to be prescribed to adult patients age 18 years and older who are obese (BMI of at least 30 kg/m^2) or who have a BMI of at least 27 kg/m^2 and have one related comorbidity (e.g., high blood pressure, T2DM, elevated cholesterol) (Novo Nordisk A/S 2014). It is contraindicated in patients who are pregnant or breastfeeding, and in patients with a history or family history of certain thyroid cancers. Patients should be monitored closely for any signs of thyroid tumors, pancreatitis, acute gallbladder disease, hypoglycemia, and kidney problems.

Notable nutrition-related side effects include, but are not limited to (Novo Nordisk A/S 2014):

- Nausea and vomiting
- Diarrhea or constipation
- Hypoglycemia

- Fatigue
- Headache
- Dizziness

Benzphetamine

Benzphetamine, or Didrex® (Pharmacia and Upjohn Company, Pfizer) (National Institutes of Health, National Library of Medicine 2011), is a prescription-only weight loss drug that works as an anorectic by suppressing the patient's appetite. As the name might imply, benzphetamine is pharmacologically and chemically similar to amphetamine. Although the amphetamine class of drugs can be used to treat obesity, these drugs can be highly addictive. As a result, benzphetamine is considered a controlled substance by the Drug Enforcement Agency and should only be used as prescribed for a limited duration.

Didrex comes in a tablet form and should be used as monotherapy (National Institutes of Health, National Library of Medicine 2011). Prior to starting this medication, clinicians should ensure that the patient is not taking any other anorectic medications, including herbal supplements. The therapeutic dose of Didrex ranges from 25 to 50 mg, one to three times daily, and clinicians should start with low doses and titrate accordingly.

This medication is contraindicated in patients younger than 12 years and in women who are pregnant or who may become pregnant. It is also contraindicated in women who are breastfeeding (National Institutes of Health, National Library of Medicine 2011). Valvular heart disease and pulmonary hypertension have been noted as rare but potential side effects of anorectic medications; therefore, patients with some cardiac-related conditions (e.g., arteriosclerosis, cardiovascular disease, and moderate to severe hypertension), glaucoma, and hyperthyroidism should avoid taking this medication. Clinicians should also avoid prescribing this medication to patients with a history of or at risk for substance abuse.

Adverse reactions to benzphetamine include heart palpitations, increased heart rate and blood pressure, and rare instances of ischemic heart disease and cardiomyopathy (National Institutes of Health, National Library of Medicine 2011). Some patients have also reported changes in libido and overstimulation while taking benzphetamine. Additional side effects that may impact a patient's nutritional status include, but are not limited to:

- Dry mouth
- Dysgeusia
- Nausea
- Diarrhea
- Insomnia
- Dizziness

Diethylpropion

Diethylpropion is an active ingredient found in Tenuate® and Tenuate Dospan® (Lannett Company, Inc.). Similar to benzphetamine, diethylpropion is a nonepinephrine releaser that can decrease appetite (National Institutes of Health, National Library of Medicine 2012). It is available as a 25 mg tablet, which can be taken three times per day 1 hour before a meal, or it is also available as a 75 mg extended release tablet, which only has to be taken once daily (National Institutes of Health, National Library of Medicine 2010).

The chemical structure of diethylpropion is similar to that of amphetamine, thus making the contraindications similar to those seen with benzphetamine. Diethylpropion is a schedule IV controlled substance, and some patients have developed a psychological dependence on the drug. Patients should only be prescribed diethylpropion for a limited duration (i.e., a few weeks) and should be weaned appropriately at the end of the course.

Nutrition-related side effects of and adverse reactions to diethylpropion are similar to those seen with benzphetamine. In addition, general malaise, abdominal discomfort and gastrointestinal distrurbances, menstrual upset, and muscle pain have also been reported (National Institutes of Health, National Library of Medicine 2010).

Combination Drugs

Phentermine and Topiramate

The weight loss drug commonly known as Qsymia (VIVUS, Inc.) (VIVUS, Inc. 2015) is made up of two prescription medications, phentermine and topiramate. Phentermine is a drug that works to suppress the appetite, whereas topiramate is commonly prescribed for those with epilepsy or migraines (U.S. Department of Health and Human Services, Food and Drug Administration 2012b). Topiramate has been associated with weight loss, particularly visceral fat loss (Verrotti et al. 2011, 189–99), which makes it an appropriate medication for obesity treatment.

The phentermine and topiramate extended release capsule is recommended for patients with a BMI of at least 30 kg/m^2 or adults with a BMI of at least 27 kg/m^2 who also have one related comorbidity (e.g., high blood pressure, T2DM, elevated cholesterol) (Shin and Gadde 2013, 131). The capsules are available in four dosages, with 3.75 mg phentermine/23 mg extended release topiramate being the smallest dose, and 15 mg phentermine/92 mg extended release topiramate being the maximum dose. Prescribing clinicians should start patients on a lower dose and titrate the dose accordingly.

Patients should expect weight loss while taking this medication. If a patient has not lost 3 percent of his body weight after taking the mid-level dose for 12 weeks, the medication should either be discontinued or the dose should be increased (VIVUS, Inc. 2014). If 5 percent body weight loss is not achieved after 12 weeks on the maximum dose, then the medication regimen should be discontinued.

Similar to medications containing lorcaserin, medications containing phentermine or topiramate should be used in conjunction with a reduced calorie diet and a physical activity regimen in order to produce weight loss (VIVUS, Inc. 2014). This medication should only be used in adults, as its safety in children under 18 years is unknown. This medication should not be taken by women who are pregnant, individuals with glaucoma or thyroid problems (namely hyperthyroidism), or individuals taking MAOIs. Caution should be exercised when prescribing this medication to individuals with liver or kidney problems.

Side effects of phentermine or topiramate that may impact nutritional status include, but are not limited to (Shin and Gadde 2013, 131):

- Dysgeusia
- Constipation
- Dry mouth

- Insomnia
- Dizziness

Naltrexone and Bupropion

The combination medication composed of naltrexone and bupropion, commonly known at Contrave® (Orexigen Therapeutics, Inc., Takeda Pharmaceuticals USA, Inc.) (Orexigen Therapeutics, Inc. 2014), may be prescribed for weight loss purposes. Each extended release tablet contains 8 mg naltrexone and 90 mg bupropion. Naltrexone is an opioid antagonist and bupropion is an antidepressant, and together with diet and exercise, this combination medication can facilitate weight loss by decreasing appetite.

Contrave is contraindicated in pregnant and nursing mothers, as well as in children under the age of 18 years (Orexigen Therapeutics, Inc. 2014). It should not be prescribed for any individuals with seizure disorders, uncontrolled high blood pressure, anorexia or bulimia, or chronic opioid use. It is also contraindicated in individuals who are undergoing discontinuation of alcohol, barbiturates, and antiepileptic drugs and who are taking MAOIs.

Patients who are prescribed this combination drug should have their blood pressure, heart rate, and blood sugars closely monitored (Orexigen Therapeutics, Inc. 2014). The medication should be discontinued if the patient begins showing symptoms of suicidal behavior or depression. Contrave may interact with several other medications, thus making it critically important that clinicians inventory all of the medications and supplements a patient is taking prior to prescribing this medication.

Nutrition-related adverse reactions to this medication include (Orexigen Therapeutics, Inc. 2014):

- Nausea and vomiting
- Constipation
- Dry mouth
- Diarrhea
- Insomnia

Summary

A variety of drugs have been approved by FDA to assist with weight loss in overweight and obese patients. Although these medications do have side effects that must be considered, they can assist in improving weight status and in lowering the risk of weight-related diseases when combined with diet and exercise.

References

Arena Pharmaceuticals GmbH. 2014. "Belviq (Lorcaserin HCl) CIV—Proven Weight Loss with Lasting Impact, Important Safety Information." www.belviqhcp.com/?utm_source=bing&utm_medium=cpc&utm_term=belvique&utm_campaign=BS%2B-%2BMisspellings_EX (accessed June 29, 2015).

Arena Pharmaceuticals GmbH. 2014. "Belviq(R) (Lorcaserin HCl) CIV—Consumer." www.belviq.com/?gclid=CKP94JadjscCFdAXHwodOOMEHw (accessed June 29, 2015).

Genentech Inc., A Member of the Roche Group. 2012. "Xenical Prescribing Information." www.gene.com/download/pdf/xenical_prescribing.pdf (accessed June 30, 2015).

Genentech Inc., A Member of the Roche Group. 2013. "Xenical.Com Home." www.xenical.com/xenical/ (accessed June 30, 2015).

GlaxoSmithKline, plc. 2013. "Healthy Weight Loss—Alli." www.myalli.com (accessed June 30, 2015).

Guerciolini, R. 1997. "Mode of Action of Orlistat." *International Journal of Obesity and Related Metabolic Disorders: Journal of the International Association for the Study of Obesity* 21, Suppl. 3, pp. S12–23.

National Institutes of Health, National Library of Medicine. 2010. "DailyMed - Diethylpropion Hydrochloride Tablet." Last modified April 2010, http://dailymed.nlm.nih.gov/dailymed/drugInfo.cfm?id=17823 (accessed July 2, 2015).

National Institutes of Health, National Library of Medicine. 2011. "DailyMed - DIDREX - Benzphetamine Hydrochloride Tablet." Last modified February 2011, http://dailymed.nlm.nih.gov/dailymed/drugInfo.cfm?id=38067 (accessed 2015).

National Institutes of Health, National Library of Medicine. 2012. "Diethylpropion: MedlinePlus Drug Information." Last modified November 20, 2012, www.nlm.nih.gov/medlineplus/druginfo/meds/a682037.html#brand-name-1 (accessed July 2, 2015).

National Institutes of Health, National Library of Medicine. 2013. "Lorcaserin: MedlinePlus Drug Information." Last modified May 15, www.nlm.nih.gov/medlineplus/druginfo/meds/a613014.html (accessed June 29, 2015).

National Institutes of Health, National Library of Medicine. 2015. "Phentermine: MedlinePlus Drug Information." Last modified January 15, www.nlm.nih.gov/medlineplus/druginfo/meds/a682187.html (accessed August 3, 2015).

Novo Nordisk A/S. 2014. "Saxenda Prescribing Information." Last modified December 2014, www.novo-pi.com/saxenda.pdf (accessed June 30, 2015).

Novo Nordisk A/S. 2015a. "Saxenda (R) (Liraglutide [rDNA Origin] Injection) Official Product Site." Last modified April 2015, www.saxenda.com (accessed June 30, 2015).

Novo Nordisk A/S. 2015b. "Victoza (R) (Liraglutide [rDNA Origin] Injection) Official Product Site." Last modified July 2015, www.victoza.com (accessed July 15, 2015).

Orexigen Therapeutics, Inc. 2014. "Contrave (R) (Naltrexone HCl and Bupropion HCl) Extended-Release Tablets: Prescribing Information." Last modified September 2014, http://general.takedapharm.com/content/file.aspx?filetypecode=CONTRAVEPI&cacheRandomizer=d34d0070-5750-4d29-b5ba-ec214eb7e382 (accessed June 19, 2015).

Shin, J.H., and K.M. Gadde. 2013. "Clinical Utility of Phentermine/Topiramate (Qsymia™) Combination for the Treatment of Obesity." *Diabetes, Metabolic Syndrome and Obesity: Targets and Therapy* 6, p. 131. doi:10.2147/dmso.s43403

Smith, S.R., N.J. Weissman, C.M. Anderson, M. Sanchez, E. Chuang, S. Stubbe, H. Bays, and W.R. Shanahan. 2010. "Multicenter, Placebo-Controlled Trial of Lorcaserin for Weight Management." *New England Journal of Medicine* 363, no. 3, pp. 245–56. doi:10.1056/nejmoa0909809

Teva Pharmaceuticals USA. 2014. "Adipex-P(R) (Phentermine HCl)," Mexico, MO. Last modified 2014, www.adipex.com (accessed .August 3, 2015).

U.S. Department of Health and Human Services, Food and Drug Administration. 2010. "FDA Drug Safety Communication: Completed Safety Review of Xenical/Alli (Orlistat) and Severe Liver Injury." Last modified May 26, www.fda.gov/Drugs/DrugSafety/PostmarketDrugSafetyInformationforPatientsandProviders/ucm213038.htm (accessed June 30, 2015).

U.S. Department of Health and Human Services, Food and Drug Administration. 2012a. "FDA Approves Belviq to Treat Some Overweight or Obese Adults." Last modified June 27, www.fda.gov/NewsEvents/Newsroom/PressAnnouncements/ucm309993.htm (accessed June 29, 2015).

U.S. Department of Health and Human Services, Food and Drug Administration. 2012b. "Medications Target Long-Term Weight Control." Last modified July 2012, www.fda.gov/downloads/ForConsumers/ConsumerUpdates/UCM312391.pdf (accessed June 30, 2015).

U.S. Department of Health and Human Services, Food and Drug Administration. 2014. "FDA Approves Weight-Management Drug Saxenda." Last modified December 23, www.fda.gov/NewsEvents/Newsroom/PressAnnouncements/ucm427913.htm (accessed June 30, 2015).

Verrotti, A., A. Scaparrotta, S. Agostinelli, S. Di Pillo, F. Chiarelli, and S. Grosso. 2011. "Topiramate-Induced Weight Loss: A Review." *Epilepsy Research* 95, no. 3, pp. 189–99. doi:10.1016/j.eplepsyres.2011.05.014

VIVUS, Inc. 2014. "Qysmia (R) Prescribing Information." Last modified October 2014, https://qsymia.com/patient/include/media/pdf/prescribing-information.pdf (accessed June 30, 2015).

VIVUS, Inc. 2015. "Qysmia (Phentermine and Topiramate Extended-Release) Capsules." Last modified 2015, https://qsymia.com (accessed August 3, 2015).

CHAPTER 11

Weight Loss Intervention: Weight Loss Surgery

In some cases, it may be appropriate for a patient to undergo weight loss, or bariatric, surgery in order to achieve a more desirable body weight. In the United States, ~193,000 weight loss surgeries were performed in 2014 alone (American Society for Metabolic and Bariatric Surgery 2015), a number that has been on the rise over the years. In this chapter, the indications for weight loss surgery and the pre- and postoperative nutritional management of these surgical patients will be explored, and four types of weight loss surgery will be discussed.

Surgical Criteria

Patients seeking weight loss surgery should meet specific criteria before undergoing a procedure. Adult patients should meet one of the following criteria (Mechanick 2013):

- Have a body mass index (BMI) ≥40 kg/m^2 without coexisting medical conditions, or
- Have a BMI ≥35 kg/m^2 and at least one obesity-related comorbidity (e.g., type 2 diabetes, hyperlipidemia, or hypertension).

Adult patients who have a BMI between 30 and 34.9 kg/m^2 may also be considered as candidates for weight loss surgery; however, the current evidence supporting the health benefits of this recommendation remains inconclusive (Mechanick 2013).

Like adults, young patients can also reap health benefits from weight loss surgery (Daniels 2005; Garcia 2006; Inge 2006); however, the surgical criteria for pediatric patients are different from that of adults. First, because children are still growing, it is not appropriate for a pediatric patient to undergo surgery until he has reached physical maturity (or 95 percent of his adult stature) (Pratt 2009). As such, weight loss surgery is only appropriate for adolescents.

Second, the BMI cut points for adolescents is also different than adults. Adolescent patients should meet one of the following criteria (Pratt 2009):

- Have a BMI ≥35 kg/m^2 and at least one major obesity-related comorbidity (e.g., type 2 diabetes, moderate to severe sleep apnea, severe nonalcoholic steatohepatitis), or
- Have a BMI ≥40 kg/m^2 and at least one other comorbidity (e.g., hypertension, dyslipidemia).

In all cases, a risk–benefit analysis should be conducted prior to the patient undergoing surgery. This analysis should include the risks of leaving obesity untreated as well as potential surgical complications. Informed consent (and for pediatric patients, parental consent) should always be obtained prior to the procedure.

Preoperative Care

Regardless of the patient's age, preoperative care should include three major components: medical clearance, nutritional counseling, and psychological evaluation.

Medical Clearance

In most cases, weight loss surgery is an elective, yet major, procedure with potential risks and complications that should be minimized. As such, it is imperative that all surgical candidates be medically cleared by an attending or primary care physician prior to the procedure.

Elements of medical clearance will vary based upon the patient's health status and current health conditions. In patients with type 2 diabetes, there is a positive association between preoperative glycemic control and postoperative remission of diabetes (Hall 2010); therefore, one of the elements of preoperative medical clearance is to achieve good blood sugar control. Glycemic control for patients without complications includes (1) a Hemoglobin A1C value of no more than 6.5 to 7.0 percent, (2) a fasting blood glucose value of no more than 110 mg/dL, or (3) a 2 hour postprandial blood glucose of no more than 140 mg/dL (Mechanick 2013). For patients with diabetes-related complications, preoperative glycemic targets may be more liberal (e.g., Hemoglobin A1C up to 8.0 percent); however, clinical judgement should be exercised when evaluating those patients with uncontrolled diabetes.

Prior to surgery, medical clearance for patients with known cardiovascular disease should include a formal cardiology consult (Mechanick 2013). For patients without cardiovascular disease, noninvasive cardiac testing (i.e., electrocardiogram) should be sufficient for preoperative clearance. All patients should have a fasting lipid panel obtained during the medical clearance process, and abnormal findings should prompt dietary intervention as appropriate.

Fertility and pregnancy are two elements of medical clearance that should be discussed thoroughly with female patients. Women of childbearing age who are considering weight loss surgery should be advised against getting pregnant for at least 12 to 18 months postoperatively (Mechanick 2013). In addition, clinicians should also warn women with polycystic ovarian syndrome (PCOS) that fertility can be greatly increased after weight loss surgery (Beard 2008; Mechanick 2013) and that they may find it easier to get pregnant.

Other elements of the preoperative medical clearance process will depend on the patient's medical history. For example, if a patient has a history of lung disease or abnormal sleep patterns (which could indicate sleep apnea), a formal pulmonary evaluation should take place (Mechanick 2013). Similarly, if a patient has a history of gastrointestinal (GI) problems, a gastroenterologist should be consulted and relevant GI tests should be performed before undergoing surgery.

Just as with most preoperative protocols, laboratory tests should be obtained as part of the medical clearance process. Box 11.1 contains a list of laboratory values that could be evaluated prior to surgery.

Box 11.1 Preoperative labwork (list is not exhaustive)

Medical labs:

Androgens (if PCOS is present or suspected)
Blood typing
CBC
Diabetes tests (Hemoglobin A1C) (if diabetes is present or suspected)
Fasting blood glucose
Fasting lipid panel
Kidney function tests
Liver function tests
Prothrombin time or INR (international normalized ratio)
Thyroid stimulating hormone (TSH) (if thyroid disease is present or suspected)
Urine analysis

Nutrition-specific labs:

25-vitmain D
Folic acid
Iron panel
Vitamin A (optional)
Vitamin B12
Vitamin E (optional)

Source: Mechanick (2013).

Nutritional Counseling

Prior to undergoing weight loss surgery, patients should receive extensive nutrition counseling from a Registered Dietitian Nutritionist (RDN) who has training in pre- and post-weight loss surgical diets.

Preoperative nutrition counseling should start with a full nutritional assessment (Aills 2008). While the main components of nutritional assessment were discussed in Chapter 4, additional considerations specific to these presurgical patients include a full review of the patient's weight history, inclusive of previous weight loss attempts. Many patients who are candidates for weight loss surgery will have tried to lose weight in the past. The clinician should note what successes and failures the patient has had, and help the patient to identify current barriers to weight loss. These barriers should be adequately addressed to ensure that they do not impede successful surgical outcomes and should be documented in the patient's medical record for follow-up discussions.

In some cases, it may be advantageous for the patient to lose weight before having the weight loss surgery. Preoperative energy restriction may reduce body weight and liver size in morbidly obese patients (Fris 2004) and thereby ease the complexity of surgery (Edholm 2011). Preoperative weight loss can also help achieve better presurgical glycemic control and potentially improve postoperative outcomes. Nutritional guidance on an energy-restricted diet may be incorporated into the preoperative nutrition counseling session; however, the clinician should ensure that the patient does not put himself at risk of malnutrition while following the restrictive diet.

Preoperative nutritional counseling should include a thorough review of the patient's nutritional labs. As noted in Box 11.1, patients should have preoperative labs obtained in order to identify any potential nutritional deficiencies. As much as possible, the nutritional deficiencies should be corrected prior to surgery in order to optimize postsurgical outcomes. In some cases, patients may need to begin nutritional supplementation with a multivitamin plus minerals while in the preoperative state; however, this need should be determined by the clinician.

In cases where the patient's metabolic or lipid panels are abnormal, preoperative nutritional counseling may include a review of healthy eating principles to optimize glycemic and lipid control. Therapeutic diets (e.g., controlled carbohydrate diets, low saturated, and trans fat diets) may be prescribed by the clinician in order to optimize diet-related medical conditions and minimize the impact of these conditions on postsurgical outcomes.

As part of the preoperative nutritional counseling sessions, clinicians should review the postoperative diet. This will prepare the patient for what he will and will not be able to eat following the procedure and will help him to mentally prepare for the dietary changes necessary to achieve optimal weight loss. These dietary changes will be discussed in detail later in this chapter.

At this point in the preoperative nutrition counseling session(s), it is important for the clinician to address any resistance or hesitations the patient may express. If the patient states that he feels unsure about undergoing the surgery or following the postoperative diet plan, the clinician should take the time to explore these feelings. Although it is normal for some patients to express minor concerns, patients who are clearly unwilling to follow the prescribed postoperative diet are not suitable candidates for the surgery and should not receive clearance.

Psychological Evaluation

Before receiving clearance for weight loss surgery, patients should undergo a psychological-behavioral evaluation (Mechanick 2013). Such an evaluation may identify clinically significant psychological disturbances that can impede surgical success (e.g., binge eating disorder). The evaluation may also help the clinician better refine the postoperative plan to ensure that the patient's mental health needs are met.

Patients who are found to exhibit addictive or impulsive behaviors (e.g., binge eating disorder, substance abuse, and dependence) should be referred for a formal mental health evaluation (Mechanick 2013). Credentialed psychological clinicians should then be in charge of determining if the patient is appropriate for surgery. In addition, patients who are found to regularly use tobacco should be advised to stop at least 6 weeks prior to surgery because poor surgical outcomes associated with tobacco use and smoking (Felix 2008; Gravante 2007; Gupta 2012).

Clinicians performing the preoperative psychological evaluation should be aware that weight loss surgical candidates have been shown to present themselves in an overly favorable way (Ambwani 2013), which may not fully reflect their true psychological state. As such, clinicians should be cautious when performing the psychological-behavioral evaluation to ensure that the assessment is accurate.

Types of Weight Loss Surgical Procedures

Over the past several decades, the types of weight loss surgeries available to patients have evolved (Deitel 2002). In 2014, 51.7 percent of the weight loss surgeries performed in the United States were laproscopic sleeve gastrectomy (LSG), although 26.8 percent were Roux-en-Y gastric bypass (RYGB) procedures and another 9.5 percent were laparoscopic adjustable gastric banding (LAGB) procedures (American Society for Metabolic and Bariatric Surgery 2015). The following sections will discuss these three procedures, how they accomplish weight loss, and the advantages and disadvantages of each procedure.

Laproscopic Sleeve Gastrectomy

The LSG is the most commonly performed weight loss surgery. In this 60 to 90 minute procedure (U.S. National Library of Medicine, National Institutes of Health 2013), the patient's stomach is sectioned and stapled vertically to create a tube-shaped pouch. The new pouch, or sleeve, is only ~15 percent of the size of the original stomach, and the remaining portion of the stomach is removed. Because the new stomach, or sleeve, can only hold ~129 cc (4.4 oz) of fluid at a time (Yehoshua 2008), food and beverage intake is greatly reduced. This limits the number of calories a patient consumes, creating a caloric deficit and inducing weight loss.

There are several reasons the LSG is a preferred method of weight loss surgery. First, this surgery keeps most of the gastrointestinal tract (e.g., esophageal and pyloric sphincters, the small and large intestines) intact and does not require a rerouting of food along the digestive tract. Second, the surgery occurs with minimal invasiveness (i.e., it is not an open bariatric surgery), and after the surgery, the body does not have to retain any foreign objects (as opposed to the gastric band procedure, which requires a device to permanently remain in the body).

Because the LSG requires the resection of a large portion of the stomach, patients will experience desirable changes in gut hormones. In particular, LSG patients experience decreases in ghrelin (Langer 2005), the hormone associated with hunger. As a result, LSG patients are typically less hungry and eat fewer calories, a state that can lead to significant weight loss. In fact, long-term studies of patients who have undergone LSG demonstrate that patients can lose >50 percent of their excess body weight (Himpens 2010, 219) after having the procedure.

Although there are many benefits to the LSG, this procedure does involve some risks. Potential complications and side effects should be acknowledged and discussed with the patient prior to surgery. Given that the procedure's target organ is the stomach, injury to the stomach can occur during the procedure. Stomach ulcers and gastritis have also been observed in patients who have previously had an LSG procedure (U.S. National Library of Medicine, National Institutes of Health). Because the procedure involves a significant reduction in stomach volume, heartburn, and gastroesophageal reflux have been reported in some patients postoperatively; however, these conditions may be mitigated intraoperatively using specific surgical techniques (Daes 2012). Other potential complications include leakage from the site of stapling, vomiting, abdominal scarring, and vitamin deficiencies (U.S. National Library of Medicine, National Institutes of Health 2013).

Roux-en-Y Gastric Bypass

The second most common weight loss surgery performed in the United States is RYGB. This procedure, which can take 2 to 4 hours to complete, involves two major steps (U.S. National Library of Medicine, National Institutes of Health 2014). In the first step, the stomach is reduced to a small pouch that holds about 1 oz of fluid (i.e., the size of a walnut). In the second step, the jejunum is resected and connected to the end of the newly created pouch. As a result of these two steps, the new digestive tract bypasses a large portion of the stomach and duodenum and, instead, food will travel from the small pouch directly into the jejunum.

After a patient undergoes RYGB, weight loss occurs via two mechanisms. First, the newly created pouch has such a small volume that the patient can only consume small amounts food at a time. This limits the patient's caloric intake and facilitates a fairly rapid weight loss. Second, RYGB rearranges the gastrointestinal tract so that food no longer passes through the duodenum. Because this region of the gastrointestinal tract is typically where nutrients are absorbed, patients who undergo RYGB may have less absorption of these nutrients and the resulting calories. This can also facilitate weight loss.

Patients who elect to have RYGB typically have long-term success with weight loss and weight maintenance. In some cases, patients have been able to lose up to 80 percent of their excess body weight after undergoing RYGB (Wittgrove 2000). Similar to changes observed in post-LSG patients, patients who have RYGB also experience favorable changes in gut hormone levels. Decreases in ghrelin (Korner 2005) and increases in peptide YY (Karamanakos 2008), both which reduce appetite and promote weight loss, have been observed in patients who have undergone RYGB.

Because the RYGB procedure is more complex than LSG, there may be a greater risk for complications (American Society for Metabolic and Bariatric Surgery 2015). Wound infections, incisional hernias, and anastomotic leaks have been previously described in patients who have undergone this surgery (DeMaria 2002). In addition, blood clots, heart attack, and strokes have also been noted as potential risks to the surgery (U.S. National Library of Medicine, National Institutes of Health 2014).

Given that nature of the surgery, patients who have undergone RYGB are at higher risk of developing nutritional deficiencies than those who undergo other weight loss surgeries that do not require a bypass of the duodenum. Many nutrients get absorbed in duodenum; thus those who have RYGB may not absorb sufficient amounts of these nutrients and may become deficient. Clinicians should monitor patients for signs of nutritional deficiencies, including those of vitamin B12, iron, folate, and calcium (American Society for Metabolic and Bariatric Surgery n.d.).

Laparoscopic Adjustable Gastric Banding

While less common than LSG and RYGB, LAGB is another surgery performed for weight loss purposes. In this procedure, an adjustable band is placed around the top of the stomach. The band is then inflated with saline, and as the band inflates, it squeezes the stomach and creates a small pouch below the esophageal sphincter. This new pouch will empty into the remainder of the stomach, and the rate at which this emptying occurs will be determined by the tightness of the band. The band can be tightened and loosened by injecting saline into a tube through a portal placed under the skin.

Just as with the other weight loss surgeries, the new pouch created by LAGB is much smaller than a normal stomach. As such, the patient should only consume small amounts of food at a time. In addition, the tightness of the band will determine how quickly food passes from the pouch into the remainder of the stomach. When the band is tight, this process happens slowly, making the patient feel fuller for a long period of time after eating. As a result, the patient is less likely to eat frequently and will consume fewer calories.

The main advantage of LAGB is that this procedure does not permanently alter the stomach. Although this procedure requires that a band be placed around the stomach, this band can be surgically removed at any time if needed. The procedure is also quicker to perform than the other weight loss surgeries, and in some cases, the procedure can even be performed on an outpatient basis. LAGB has the lowest rate of postoperative complications among the various types of weight loss surgeries, and patients who have this procedure are at low risk of developing nutrient deficiencies (American Society for Metabolic and Bariatric Surgery n.d.).

For some patients, however, the disadvantages of having LAGB will outweigh the benefits. The first major disadvantage of having LAGB is that, compared to other forms of weight loss surgery, this procedure may yield a slower rate of weight loss immediately after surgery (Academy of Nutrition and Dietetics 2009; American Society for Metabolic and Bariatric Surgery n.d.). Given that weight loss is one of the main goals of having this type of procedure, many patients will opt for another procedure simply because they want to see more rapid results. It should be noted, however, that one systematic review has shown that long-term weight loss among those undergoing LAGB is quite similar to those who had RYGB (O'Brien 2013).

Another disadvantage to LAGB is that a foreign device must remain in the body after surgery. Although this may not immediately be a problem, over time the band may develop mechanical problems, or it may slip or erode (Himpens 2011). Among all patients who have weight loss surgery, the highest rate of reoperation is among those who have LAGB

(American Society for Metabolic and Bariatric Surgery n.d.), and this is also a major disadvantage to this procedure.

Other Weight Loss Procedures

In addition to the three procedures previously discussed, a small percentage of patients may elect to have a procedure known as biliopancreatic diversion with duodenal switch (BDB/DS). Although this procedure is associated with dramatic weight loss, it also has a very high rate of complications, and patients who undergo this procedure are at much higher risk of developing nutritional deficiencies (American Society for Metabolic and Bariatric Surgery n.d.). Less than 1 percent of weight loss surgeries in the United States are BPD/DS (American Society for Metabolic and Bariatric Surgery 2015), and this procedure is not recommended for adolescents (Pratt 2009).

It is also possible for patients to undergo one type of weight loss surgery, then later undergo another type of surgery. For example, a patient may first have LAGB, then decide to have RYGB performed at a later date. This progression of surgeries typically starts with LAGB because this surgery is reversible; however, having multiple surgeries is not typically recommended unless a patient is unsuccessful with losing a significant amount of excess weight a year or more after the first procedure.

Postoperative Nutrition Therapy

Patients who have undergone weight loss surgery will need to follow a strict diet immediately after the procedure. Ideally, diet orders and nutritional guidance should be provided by a trained RDN who can explain the nutrition principles to the patient and ensure that the patient understands the importance of following these principles.

Clear and Full Liquids

Within 24 hours of the procedure, a bariatric clear liquid diet is typically initiated for the postoperative patient (Mechanick 2013). All liquids should be free of sugar, calories, and carbonation, and they should not contain caffeine or alcohol (Academy of Nutrition and Dietetics

2015). Water, decaffeinated coffee and tea, and sugar-free flavored waters are all appropriate for this dietary phase. Sugar-free gelatin, sugar-free popsicles (25 kcal or less per popsicle), clear broths, and low-sugar vegetable juices (e.g., tomato juice) may also be consumed. Sugary liquids, gelatin, and popsicles should be avoided because their high sugar content may cause dumping syndrome, which leads to dehydration. These products are also high in empty calories and ingesting them would essentially defeat the purpose of the surgery. As such, sugary liquids and foods should be avoided by these postoperative patients.

As soon as medically feasible, the patient's diet should be advanced to include full liquids. The bariatric full liquid diet is considered nutritionally adequate because it can be formulated to include all essential nutrients, including protein. The protein needs of a weight loss surgery patient will vary; however, 60 g/day or 1.5 g of protein per kilogram of ideal body weight is usually adequate (Mechanick 2013). Some patients may have higher protein needs (up to 2.1 g of protein per kilogram of ideal body weight [Mechanick 2013]), but this should be assessed by an RDN on an individual basis.

Similar to the clear liquid diet, the full liquid diet for postoperative patients should be low in sugar. Protein-containing products such as milk, soy milk, yogurt (smooth, without chunks), and protein shakes are appropriate for this diet; however, they should contain minimal (if any) added sugars. To keep the diet low in calories and minimize potential gastrointestinal distress, these full liquid products should also be low in fat. As such, all milk products should be non- or low-fat (1 percent). Sugar-free puddings, which are also appropriate for full liquid diets, should be made with nonfat or low-fat milk.

Most patients will want to add protein shakes to the diets once they begin full liquids. Protein shakes can be purchased commercially, or they can be made by the patient. If the patient is making the shake, they should be instructed to use nonfat or low-fat milk or water as the base, then add low-sugar protein powder and flavoring extracts (e.g., almond, vanilla, or peppermint extract) if desired. Patients should avoid adding fruit or fruit juice to flavor these shakes because the sugar content may become too high. Patients can also make protein shakes by mixing no-sugar-added instant breakfast powders with nonfat or low-fat milk.

Patients will need to follow a liquids-only diet for ~2 weeks after their weight loss surgery. During this time, women will need to consume ~24 oz of clear liquids and 24 oz of full liquids, and men will need to consume ~30 oz of clear liquids and 30 oz of full liquids (Academy of Nutrition and Dietetics 2015). Patients should be instructed to sip the fluids slowly and avoid using straws. This will keep them from ingesting extra air and feeling bloated.

Supplementation

To avoid developing a nutritional deficiency, patients must also take several vitamins and minerals after the surgery. For patients who underwent LSG or RYGB, two chewable multivitamins with minerals (e.g., a children's "complete" supplement with iron, thiamin, and folic acid) (Academy of Nutrition and Dietetics 2015; Mechanick 2013) should be taken about an hour after breakfast. Two chewable calcium supplements should be taken later in the day at separate times (e.g., one supplement at lunch and the other supplement at dinner) so the total daily calcium intake is 1,200 to 1,500 mg (Mechanick 2013). A daily vitamin D supplement of at least 3,000 International Units, should be consumed, as should one sublingual vitamin B12 supplement. For patients who underwent Laparoscopic Gastric Bypass (LGB), a similar vitamin and mineral supplementation schedule is prescribed. These patients need the same calcium and vitamin D as those who had LSG and RYGB; however, LGB patients will only need to take one chewable multivitamin with minerals each day, and they may not need the vitamin B12 supplement.

A sample menu showing when the postoperative RYGB patient should consume clear and full liquids as well as the vitamin and mineral supplements is seen in Box 11.2.

Box 11.2 Sample liquid menu for male patient who recently had RYGB

Breakfast, 06:30:

10 oz of protein shake (made with skim milk and no-sugar-added instant breakfast powder)

Midmorning, 08:30–10:30:

Slowly consume 10 oz of water flavored with lemon

Take 2 chewable multivitamins with minerals and 1 vitamin D supplement

Lunch, 11:00:

4 oz of sugar-free pudding made with skim milk

Take 1 chewable calcium supplement and 1 vitamin B12 supplement

Early afternoon, 13:30:

6 oz of light Greek yogurt

Late afternoon, 14:30–16:30:

Slowly consume 10 oz of sugar-free, calorie-free sports drink

Dinner, 18:00:

10 oz of commercially prepared low-sugar protein shake

Take 1 chewable calcium supplement

Late evening, 19:30–21:30:

4 oz of sugar-free gelatin

Slowly consume 6 oz of water

Bariatric Soft Diet

Approximately 2 weeks following the surgery, patients may begin introducing soft-consistency solid foods (Academy of Nutrition and Dietetics, Nutrition Care Manual 2015). These foods should be protein-rich and should be introduced in very small amounts. During the first week of this diet, all foods should be extremely soft and moist. Examples of these foods include scrambled eggs and egg whites, tofu, cottage cheese, and well-cooked beans and lentils. Other soft foods such as cooked vegetables, soft fruits, and animal proteins (e.g., fish, chicken) may be introduced after 1 week of starting the soft diet.

Once patients begin the soft diet, they should be encouraged to chew their foods thoroughly. Because the stomach muscle is still recovering from the surgery, its grinding capacity remains limited; thus food must be thoroughly chewed before swallowing.

Patients should continue sipping the same clear liquids they were permitted during the clear liquid phase of their postsurgical diet; however, liquids should be consumed no sooner than 30 minutes after they have finished their meal (Mechanick 2013). This will ensure that the patient receives adequate protein before he fills up on liquids. Patients will also need to continue avoiding all starchy foods (e.g., bread, pasta, rice, and cereal) because these foods have minimal protein and cause the patient to feel extremely full and uncomfortable.

Patients who are following the soft diet will end up consuming 3 to 5 small meals throughout the day. They should continue following their vitamin and mineral regimen, and they should also continue sipping on low-calorie clear liquids to stay hydrated. A sample menu for this soft diet is seen in Box 11.3.

Box 11.3 ***Sample soft diet menu for female who recently had LSG***

Breakfast, 06:30:

2 scrambled egg whites
(30 minutes after meal, can begin to sip on clear liquids)

(*Continued*)

(*Continued*)

Midmorning, 08:30–10:30:

Slowly consume 12 oz of water flavored with lemon
Take 2 chewable multivitamins with minerals and 1 vitamin D supplement

Lunch, 11:00:

1/2 cup low-fat cottage cheese
Take 1 chewable calcium supplement and 1 vitamin B12 supplement
(30 minutes after meal, can begin to sip on clear liquids)

Afternoon, 14:00–17:00:

8 oz protein shake
After eating yogurt, slowly consume 12 oz of sugar-free lemonade

Dinner, 18:00:

1/2–3/4 cup tofu flavored with soy sauce
Take 1 chewable calcium supplement
(30 minutes after meal, can begin to sip on clear liquids)

Late evening, 19:30–21:30:

6 oz light Greek yogurt
(30 minutes after, slowly consume 12 oz of decaffeinated tea)

Long-Term Diet

Once a postsurgical patient has been following the soft diet for several weeks, he can begin slowly transitioning to a full food diet. Nonetheless, the patient should be reminded that his stomach is still much smaller than it was pre-surgery; thus portion sizes should remain small and food should be thoroughly chewed. This will also help the patient to control his caloric intake and will promote weight loss.

At meals, patients should continue eating protein-containing foods before they eat other foods. They should have at least five servings of fruits and vegetables each day (Mechanick 2013) and should avoid refined starches, carbonated beverages, and other empty calorie foods and beverages.

Patients should also continue with the same vitamin and mineral supplementation regimen they followed immediately after surgery. Clinicians will need to monitor patients for their nutritional status by checking biochemical indicators such as iron, 25-hydroxyvitamin D, and vitamin A. Clinicians may also want to monitor bone mineral density using dual-energy x-ray absorptiometry (DXA). Patients who are undergoing RYBG and BPD/DS should have DXA performed at baseline before the surgery and 2 years after the surgery to detect for osteoporosis (Mechanick 2013).

Summary

Weight loss surgery is a viable option for obese patients who have not been able to lose weight through diet and exercise alone. Although the surgery is a more invasive and extreme measure, it can produce dramatic results and significantly lower the patient's risk of morbidity and mortality.

References

Academy of Nutrition and Dietetics. 2015. "Roux-en-Y Gastric Bypass/sleeve Gastrectomy Discharge Nutrition Therapy." www.nutritioncaremanual.org/client_ed.cfm?ncm_client_ed_id=339

Academy of Nutrition and Dietetics. 2009. "Nutrition Care Bariatric Surgery (NCBS): Weight Loss and Weight Regain Expected After Procedure (2009)." www.andeal.org/topic.cfm?menu=1406&cat=3845

Academy of Nutrition and Dietetics, Nutrition Care Manual. 2015. "Bariatric Surgery Soft Protein-Rich Foods Nutrition Therapy." www.nutritioncaremanual.org/client_ed.cfm?ncm_client_ed_id=334

Aills, L., J. Blankenship, C. Buffington, M. Furtado, J. Parrott, and Allied Health Sciences Section Ad Hoc Nutrition Committee. 2008. "ASMBS Allied Health Nutritional Guidelines for the Surgical Weight Loss Patient." *Surgery for Obesity and Related Diseases* 4, no. 5, pp. S73–108.

Ambwani, S., A.G. Boeka, J.D. Brown, T.K. Byrne, A.R. Budak, D.B. Sarwer, A.N. Fabricatore, L.C. Morey, and P.M. O'Neil. 2013. "Socially Desirable Responding by Bariatric Surgery Candidates During Psychological Assessment." *Surgery for Obesity and Related Diseases* 9, no. 2, pp. 300–5.

American Society for Metabolic and Bariatric Surgery. 2015. "Bariatric Surgery Procedures." http://asmbs.org/patients/bariatric-surgery-procedures

American Society for Metabolic and Bariatric Surgery. 2015. "Estimate of Bariatric Surgery Numbers, 2011–2014." http://asmbs.org/resources/estimate-of-bariatric-surgery-numbers

Beard, J.H., R.L. Bell, and A.J. Duffy. 2008. "Reproductive Considerations and Pregnancy After Bariatric Surgery: Current Evidence and Recommendations." *Obesity Surgery* 18, no. 8, pp. 1023–7.

Daes, J., M.E. Jimenez, N. Said, J.C. Daza, and R. Dennis. 2012. "Laparoscopic Sleeve Gastrectomy: Symptoms of Gastroesophageal Reflux Can Be Reduced by Changes in Surgical Technique." *Obesity Surgery* 22, no. 12, pp. 1874–9.

Daniels, S.R., D.K. Arnett, R.H. Eckel, S.S. Gidding, L.L. Hayman, S. Kumanyika, T.N. Robinson, B.J. Scott, S. St Jeor, and C.L. Williams. 2005. Overweight in Children and Adolescents: Pathophysiology, Consequences, Prevention, and Treatment. *Circulation* 111, no. 15, pp. 1999–2012.

Deitel, M., and S.A. Shikora. 2002. "The Development of The Surgical Treatment of Morbid Obesity." *Journal of the American College of Nutrition* 21, no. 5, pp. 365–71.

DeMaria, E.J., H.J. Sugerman, J.M. Kellum, J.G. Meador, and L.G. Wolfe. 2002. "Results of 281 Consecutive Total laparoscopic roux-en-Y Gastric Bypasses to Treat Morbid Obesity." *Annals of Surgery* 235, no. 5, p. 640, discussion 645–7.

Edholm, D., J. Kullberg, A. Haenni, F.A. Karlsson, A. Ahlström, J. Hedberg, H. Ahlström, and M. Sundbom. 2011. "Preoperative 4-Week Low-Calorie Diet Reduces Liver Volume and Intrahepatic Fat, and Facilitates Laparoscopic Gastric Bypass in Morbidly Obese." *Obesity Surgery* 21, no. 3, pp. 345–50.

Felix, E.L., J. Kettelle, E. Mobley, and D. Swartz. 2008. "Perforated Marginal Ulcers After Laparoscopic Gastric Bypass." *Surgical Endoscopy* 22, no. 10, pp. 2128–32.

Fris, R.J. 2004. "Preoperative low Energy Diet Diminishes Liver Size." *Obesity Surgery* 14, no. 9, pp. 1165–70.

Garcia, V.F., and E.J. DeMaria. 2006. "Adolescent Bariatric Surgery: Treatment Delayed, Treatment Denied, a Crisis Invited." *Obesity Surgery* 16, no. 1, pp. 1–4.

Gravante, G., A. Araco, R. Sorge, F. Araco, D. Delogu, and V. Cervelli. 2007. "Wound Infections in Post-Bariatric Patients Undergoing Body Contouring Abdominoplasty: The Role of Smoking." *Obesity Surgery* 17, no. 10, pp. 1325–31.

Gupta, P.K., H. Gupta, M. Kaushik, X. Fang, W.J. Miller, L.E. Morrow, and R. Armour-Forse. 2012. "Predictors of Pulmonary Complications After Bariatric Surgery." *Surgery for Obesity and Related Diseases* 8, no. 5, pp. 574–81.

Hall, T.C., M.G.C. Pellen, P.C. Sedman, and P.K. Jain. 2010. "Preoperative Factors Predicting Remission of Type 2Diabetes Mellitus After Roux-en-Y Gastric Bypass Surgery for Obesity." *Obesity Surgery* 20, no. 9, pp. 1245–50.

Himpens, J., G.B. Cadière, M. Bazi, M. Vouche, B. Cadière, and G. Dapri. 2011. "Long-term Outcomes of Laparoscopic Adjustable Gastric Banding." *Archives of Surgery* 146, no. 7, pp. 802–7.

Himpens, J., J. Dobbeleir, and G. Peeters. 2010. "Long-term Results of Laparoscopic Sleeve Gastrectomy for Obesity." *Annals of Surgery* 252, no. 2, pp. 319–24.

Inge, T.H. 2006. "Bariatric Surgery for Morbidly Obese Adolescents: Is There a Rationale for Early Intervention? *Growth Hormone & IGF Researc*h 16, pp. 15–9.

Karamanakos, S.N., K. Vagenas, F. Kalfarentzos, and T.K. Alexandrides. 2008. "Weight Loss, Appetite Suppression, and Changesin Fasting and Postprandial Ghrelin and Peptide-YY Levels After Roux-en-Y Gastric Bypass and Sleeve Gastrectomy: A Prospective, Double Blind Study." *Annals of Surgery* 247, no. 3, pp. 401–7.

Korner, J., M. Bessler, L.J. Cirilo, I.M. Conwell, A. Daud, N.L. Restuccia, and S.L. Wardlaw. 2005. "Effects of Roux-en-Y Gastric Bypass Surgery on Fasting and Postprandial Concentrations of Plasma Ghrelin, Peptide YY, and Insulin." *The Journal of Clinical Endocrinology & Metabolism* 90, no. 1, pp. 359–65.

Langer, F.B, M.A. Reza Hoda, A. Bohdjalian, F.X. Felberbauer, J. Zacherl, E. Wenzl, K. Schindler, A. Luger, B. Ludvik, and G. Prager. 2005. "Sleeve Gastrectomy and Gastric Banding: Effects on Plasma Ghrelin Levels." *Obesity Surgery* 15, no. 7, pp. 1024–9.

Mechanick, J.I., A. Youdim, D.B. Jones, W.T. Garvey, D.L. Hurley, M.M. McMahon, L.J. Heinberg, R. Kushner, T.D. Adams, and S. Shikora. 2013. "Clinical Practice Guidelines for the Perioperative Nutritional, Metabolic, and Nonsurgical Support of the Bariatric Surgery Patient—2013 Update: Cosponsored by American Association of Clinical Endocrinologists, the Obesity Society, and American Society for Metabolic & Bariatric Surgery." *Obesity* 21, no. S1, pp. S1–S27.

O'Brien, P.E., L. MacDonald, M. Anderson, L. Brennan, and W.A. Brown. 2013. "Long-Term Outcomes After Bariatric Surgery: Fifteen-Year follow-up of Adjustable Gastric Banding and a Systematic Review of The Bariatric Surgical Literature." *Annals of Surgery* 257, no. 1, pp. 87–94.

Pratt, J.S.A., C.M. Lenders, E.A. Dionne, A.G. Hoppin, G.L.K Hsu, T.H. Inge, D.F. Lawlor, M.F. Marino, A.F. Meyers, and J.L. Rosenblum. 2009. "Best Practice Updates for Pediatric/Adolescent Weight Loss Surgery." *Obesity* 17, no. 5, pp. 901–10.

U.S. National Library of Medicine, National Institutes of Health. 2014. "Gastric Bypass Surgery: Medline Plus Medical Encyclopedia." www.nlm.nih.gov/medlineplus/ency/article/007199.htm

U.S. National Library of Medicine, National Institutes of Health. 2013. "Vertical Sleeve Gastrectomy: Medline Plus Medical Encyclopedia." www.nlm.nih.gov/medlineplus/ency/article/007435.htm

Wittgrove, A.C., and G.W. Clark. 2000. "Laparoscopic Gastric Bypass, Roux en-Y-500 Patients: Technique and Results, with 3–60 Month Follow-Up." *Obesity Surgery* 10, no. 3, pp. 233–9.

Yehoshua, R.T., L.A. Eidelman, M. Stein, S. Fichman, A. Mazor, J. Chen, H. Bernstine, P. Singer, R. Dickman, and S.A. Shikora. 2008. "Laparoscopic Sleeve Gastrectomy—Volume and Pressure Assessment." *Obesity Surgery* 18, no. 9, pp. 1083–8.

CHAPTER 12

Physical Activity

Although the majority of this textbook has focused on the energy intake side of the energy balance equation, all weight management programs should also emphasize on the energy output (or energy expenditure) side of the equation. As discussed in Chapter 1, energy output is comprised of multiple factors (i.e., basal metabolism, physical activity, and the thermic effect of food); however, physical activity is considered to be the most significant because it is the easiest to modify. This final chapter will discuss physical activity in the context of weight management for both adult and pediatric patients.

Federal Guidelines

Just as the federal government has released general guidelines for healthy eating, it has also released general guidelines for physical activity. The science-based document, *Physical Activity Guidelines for Americans*, was released in 2008 (U.S. Department of Health and Human Services 2008), and this document makes several recommendations for American adults and children.

The *Guidelines* recommend adults avoid inactivity and aim for at least 150 minutes of moderate-intensity or 75 minutes of vigorous-intensity aerobic activity each week (U.S. Department of Health and Human Services 2008). In addition, they recommend adults perform muscle-strengthening activities for all major muscle groups (i.e., legs, hips, back, abdomen, chest, shoulders, and arms) at least 2 days each week.

For children and adolescents, the *Guidelines* recommend at least 60 minutes a day of physical activity (U.S. Department of Health and Human Services 2008). Physical activity for children is divided into three major categories: aerobic, muscle-strengthening, and bone-strengthening. According to the *Guidelines*, most of the 60 minutes each day should be spent doing moderate- or vigorous-intensity aerobic physical activities (e.g., running, dancing, and swimming), and vigorous-intensity aerobic activities should be incorporated at least 3 days each week. As part of the 60 minutes each day, children should incorporate muscle-strengthening activities (e.g., climbing and playing tug-of-war) and bone-strengthening activities (e.g., basketball and jumping rope) on 3 days each week, respectively.

Developing a Physical Activity Plan

Because many overweight and obese patients may not be physically active when they first enter a weight management program, it is important that they start an activity plan that is appropriate for their entry level of fitness. Before starting any kind of exercise regimen, patients with chronic illnesses should first receive medical clearance (U.S. Department of Health and Human Services 2008). Once they received this clearance, they should work with a clinician to develop an initial plan that incorporates enjoyable activities. This is essential for keeping a patient motivated and interested in performing the physical activities, as patients may be inclined to stop exercising if they do not enjoy the activities prescribed in their plan.

The initial physical activity plan will be modified over time as the patient becomes more fit. The amount of time spent in physical activity and the intensity of the exercises should slowly be increased to help the patient reach maximum fitness. However, when increasing the amount of time spent exercising, clinicians and their patients should discuss any potential barriers to meeting these new goals and ensure that the new plan is reasonable and achievable.

Effects on Weight Status and Body Composition

Generally speaking, physical activity and exercise has favorable effects on body composition. Among children, time spent in very high intensity activities is inversely associated with body fat and body mass index (BMI) (Abbott and Davies 2004, 285–91; Collings et al. 2013, 1020–28), and similar results are seen with BMI in adults (Ching et al. 1996). As would be expected, individuals who participate in regular physical activity may also have higher percentages of fat-free mass, including muscle mass.

Given the nature of the tissue, muscle mass is more dense and weighs more than fat mass or adipose tissue. As such, patients participating in weight management programs should be cautioned that their rate of total weight loss may be slowed as lean body mass is gained. Patients may be discouraged when their weight is not decreasing at a rapid rate; however, if they continue to exercise and gain muscle mass, they should lose inches (i.e., the circumferences of their waist, hips, arms, and legs may decrease). In some programs, clinicians will monitor these measurements in addition to the patient's body weight as a more comprehensive evaluation of the patient's progress.

Effects on Physical Health Outcomes

As previously discussed in Chapter 2, overweight and obesity are associated with a myriad of poor health outcomes. Because weight loss and an achievement of a lower weight status can eradicate many of these health risks, many patients will seek out weight management programs. Physical activity, in and of itself, can also improve health status and lower the risk of many health conditions associated with obesity.

According to the Centers for Disease Control and Prevention, physical activity alone can lower an individual's risk of many chronic health conditions (U.S. Department of Health and Human Services, Centers for Disease Control and Prevention 2015a). For adults, getting 150 minutes of moderate-intensity physical activity each week can lower the risk of cardiovascular disease and stroke, the number 1 and number 5 leading causes of death in the United States (U.S. Department of Health and Human Services, Centers for Disease Control and Prevention 2015b). A similar amount of activity (120 to 150 minutes of moderate activity each week) may also lower the risk of metabolic syndrome and type 2 diabetes mellitus. In older adults, higher amounts of exercise and activity have been associated with lower levels of undesirable inflammatory markers (Colbert et al. 2004).

Cancer risk can also be impacted by regular physical activity (U.S. Department of Health and Human Services, Centers for Disease Control and Prevention 2015a). Some studies have suggested that the risks of developing colon and lung cancer can be mitigated by physical activity. Among women, the risks of developing breast and endometrial cancers may also be lowered by regular physical activity.

Symptoms of other chronic health conditions may be improved by regular physical activity. For example, studies have demonstrated that heavier individuals are more at risk than their lower weight counterparts for developing arthritis (Voigt et al. 1994; Felson et al. 1988). The Centers for Disease Control and Prevention report that performing as little as 130 to 150 minutes of moderate-intensity, low-impact physical activity can improve pain management and quality of life in individuals with arthritis (U.S. Department of Health and Human Services, Centers for Disease Control and Prevention 2015a). In addition, the progressive loss of bone density and the risk of hip fracture, both of which increase with aging, may also be lowered by regular physical activity (U.S. Department of Health and Human Services, Centers for Disease Control and Prevention 2015a; Englund et al. 2011, 499–505; Armstrong et al. 2011, 1330–38).

Effects on Mental Health

Regular physical activity not only improves physical health; it also improves mental health. As discussed in Chapter 2, many mental health disturbances are correlated with obesity and high weight status. As such, physical activity has been proposed as a means to improve these conditions as well as to assist with weight management.

Studies have long demonstrated that physical activity can have a positive impact on symptoms of depression (Dunn, Trivedi, and O'Neal 2001). It has also been shown to improve mood states and general quality of life (Penedo and Dahn 2005). While not as effective as pharmaceutical interventions, exercise and physical activity have also been shown to help manage symptoms of anxiety as well (Carek, Laibstain, and Carek 2011).

Because of the known mental health benefits of physical activity, researchers have called on mental health providers to incorporate regular physical activity into the treatment of patients with mental health conditions (Richardson et al. 2005). Although physical activity should not be a substitute for other mental health services and pharmacotherapies, it can be beneficial and may improve patients' symptoms.

Effect on Food Intake

When a patient who was previously inactive begins an exercise routine, the amount of calories he expends will increase. Theoretically, the body may try to compensate for this additional expenditure by inducing hunger and causing the patient to ingest more calories; however, this does not appear to be the case. In fact, multiples studies have demonstrated that overweight individuals who begin an exercise program will not compensate for the additional energy expenditure by eating more calories (Donnelly et al. 2003, 1343–50; Cox et al. 2003, 107–15; Donnelly et al. 2000, 566–72; Pritchard, Nowson, and Wark 1997, 37–42) and that this desirable effect is long term.

The exact mechanism by which energy intake does not increase with higher levels of physical activity is still being explored. One study hypothesized that this could be because physical activity increases the feelings of satiety after a meal (King et al. 2009). Another study suggested that exercise induced lower levels of ghrelin, which corresponded to lower levels of hunger (Broom et al. 2007).

Summary

Physical activity has many beneficial health effects and can attenuate weight loss in patients who are overweight and obese. Patients should be encouraged to incorporate regular physical activity into their weight loss regimen and should be monitored for improvements in fitness as their regimen progresses.

References

Abbott, R.A., and P.S.W. Davies. 2004. "Habitual Physical Activity and Physical Activity Intensity: Their Relation to Body Composition in 5.0–10.5-Y-Old Children." *European Journal of Clinical Nutrition* 58, no. 2, pp. 285–91. doi:10.1038/sj.ejcn.1601780

Armstrong, M.E.G., E.A. Spencer, B.J. Cairns, E. Banks, K. Pirie, J. Green, F.L. Wright, G.K. Reeves, and V. Beral. 2011. "Body Mass Index and Physical Activity in Relation to the Incidence of Hip Fracture in Postmenopausal Women." *Journal of Bone and Mineral Research* 26, no. 6, pp. 1330–38. doi:10.1002/jbmr.315

Broom, D.R., D.J. Stensel, N.C. Bishop, S.F. Burns, and M. Miyashita. 2007. "Exercise-Induced Suppression of Acylated Ghrelin in Humans." *Journal of Applied Physiology* 102, no. 6, pp. 2165–71. doi:10.1152/japplphysiol.00759.2006

Carek, P.J., S.E. Laibstain, and S.M. Carek. 2011. "Exercise for the Treatment of Depression and Anxiety." *International Journal of Psychiatry in Medicine* 41, no. 1, pp. 15–28.

Ching, P.L., W.C. Willett, E.B. Rimm, G.A. Colditz, S.L. Gortmaker, and M.J. Stampfer. January 1996. "Activity Level and Risk of Overweight in Male Health Professionals." *American Journal of Public Health* 86, no. 1, pp. 25–30. doi:10.2105/ajph.86.1.25

Colbert, L.H., M. Visser, E.M. Simonsick, R.P. Tracy, A.B. Newman, S.B. Kritchevsky, M. Pahor, D.R. Taaffe, J. Brach, and S. Rubin. 2004. "Physical Activity, Exercise, and Inflammatory Markers in Older Adults: Findings from the Health, Aging and Body Composition Study." *Journal of the American Geriatrics Society* 52, no. 7, pp. 1098–104. doi:10.1111/j.1532-5415.2004.52307.x

Collings, P.J., S. Brage, C.L. Ridgway, N.C. Harvey, K.M. Godfrey, H.M. Inskip, C. Cooper, N.J. Wareham, and U. Ekelund. May 2013. "Physical Activity Intensity, Sedentary Time, and Body Composition in Preschoolers." *The American Journal of Clinical Nutrition* 97, no. 5, pp. 1020–28. doi:10.3945/ajcn.112.045088

Cox, K.L., V. Burke, A.R. Morton, L.J. Beilin, and I.B. Puddey. 2003. "The Independent and Combined Effects of 16 Weeks of Vigorous Exercise and Energy Restriction on Body Mass and Composition in Free-Living Overweight Men—A Randomized Controlled Trial." *Metabolism* 52, no. 1, pp. 107–15. doi:10.1053/meta.2003.50017

Donnelly, J.E., J.O. Hill, D.J. Jacobsen, J. Potteiger, D.K. Sullivan, S.L. Johnson, K. Heelan, M. Hise, P.V. Fennessey, and B. Sonko. 2003. "Effects of a 16-Month Randomized Controlled Exercise Trial on Body Weight and Composition in Young, Overweight Men and Women: The Midwest Exercise Trial." *Archives of Internal Medicine* 163, no. 11, pp. 1343–50. doi:10.1001/archinte.163.11.1343

Donnelly, J.E., D.J. Jacobsen, K.S. Heelan, R. Seip, and S. Smith. May 2000. "The Effects of 18 Months of Intermittent vs. Continuous Exercise on Aerobic Capacity, Body Weight and Composition, and Metabolic Fitness in Previously Sedentary, Moderately Obese Females." *International Journal of Obesity and Related Metabolic Disorders: Journal of the International Association for the Study of Obesity* 24, no. 5, pp. 566–72. doi:10.1038/sj.ijo.0801198

Dunn, A.L., M.H. Trivedi, and H.A. O'Neal. 2001. "Physical Activity Dose–Response Effects on Outcomes of Depression and Anxiety." *Medicine and Science in Sports and Exercise* 33, pp. S587–97. doi:10.1097/00005768-200106001-00027

Englund, U., P. Nordström, J. Nilsson, G. Bucht, U. Björnstig, G. Hallmans, O. Svensson, and U. Pettersson. 2011. "Physical Activity in Middle-Aged Women and Hip Fracture Risk: The UFO Study." *Osteoporosis International* 22, no. 2, pp. 499–505. doi:10.1007/s00198-010-1234-1

Felson, D.T., J.J. Anderson, A. Naimark, A.M. Walker, and R.F. Meenan. 1988. "Obesity and Knee Osteoarthritis: The Framingham Study." *Annals of Internal Medicine* 109, no. 1, pp. 18–24. doi:10.7326/0003-4819-109-1-18

King, N.A., P.P. Caudwell, M. Hopkins, J.R. Stubbs, E. Naslund, and J.E. Blundell. October 2009. "Dual-Process Action of Exercise on Appetite Control: Increase in Orexigenic Drive but Improvement in Meal-Induced Satiety." *The American Journal of Clinical Nutrition* 90, no. 4, pp, 921–27. doi:10.3945/ajcn.2009.27706

Penedo, F.J., and J.R. Dahn. March 2005. "Exercise and Well-Being: A Review of Mental and Physical Health Benefits Associated with Physical Activity." *Current Opinion in Psychiatry* 18, no. 2, pp. 189–93. doi:10.1097/00001504-200503000-00013

Pritchard, J.E., C.A. Nowson, and J.D. Wark. 1997. "A Worksite Program for Overweight Middle-Aged Men Achieves Lesser Weight Loss with Exercise than with Dietary Change. *Journal of the American Dietetic Association* 97, no. 1, pp. 37–42. doi:10.1016/s0002-8223(97)00015-1

Richardson, C.R., G. Faulkner, J. McDevitt, G.S. Skrinar, D.S. Hutchinson, and J.D. Piette. 2005. "Integrating Physical Activity into Mental Health Services for Persons with Serious Mental Illness." *Psychiatric Services* 56, no. 3, pp. 324–31. doi:10.1176/appi.ps.56.3.324

U.S. Department of Health and Human Services. 2008. "Physical Activity Guidelines for Americans." Available from www.health.gov/paguidelines/pdf/paguide.pdf

U.S. Department of Health and Human Services, Centers for Disease Control and Prevention. 2015a. "The Benefits of Physical Activity." www.cdc.gov/physicalactivity/basics/pa-health/index.htm

U.S. Department of Health and Human Services, Centers for Disease Control and Prevention. 2015b. "National Center for Health Statistics, Leading Causes of Death." www.cdc.gov/nchs/fastats/leading-causes-of-death.htm

Voigt, L.F., T.D. Koepsell, J. Lee Nelson, C.E. Dugowson, and J.R. Daling. 1994. "Smoking, Obesity, Alcohol Consumption, and the Risk of Rheumatoid Arthritis." *Epidemiology* 5, no. 5, pp. 525–32.

Index

Acanthosis Nigricans, 56
Acceptable macronutrient distribution range (AMDR), 95
Adipose tissue, 7
Affirmation statement, 130
AMDR. *See* Acceptable macronutrient distribution range
Amino acids, 6
Animal fats, 96
Antioxidants, 102

Bariatric soft diet, 171–172
BDB/DS. *See* Biliopancreatic diversion with duodenal switch
BED. *See* Binge eating disorder
Benzphetamine, 150–151
Biliopancreatic diversion with duodenal switch (BDB/DS), 167
Binge eating disorder (BED), 30, 31
Biochemical indicators
  cholesterol, 52–53
  c-reactive protein, 54
  glucose and associated indicators, 51–52
  reference values, 54
  uric acid, 53
Blood pressure, 55
BMI. *See* Body mass index
Body mass index (BMI)
  bed scales, 45
  children's growth charts, 43
  classifications, 45–46
  Frankfort horizontal plane, 42
  infantometer, 43
  limitation, 41
  patient's height and weight, 42
  pediatric pan scale, 44
  stadiometer, 42
  standing position, 44
  standing scale, 44
  vertical height, 43
  weight status, 42
  wheelchair scales, 45
  WHO Growth Charts, 46
Bupropion, 153

Calorie balance
  carbohydrates, 3–4
  fats, 4–5
  foods and beverage, 2
  nutrition facts label, 2
  protein, 5–6
Cancer, 15–16
Cardiovascular disease, 13–14
CDC. *See* Centers for Disease Control and Prevention
Centers for Disease Control and Prevention (CDC), 46, 47, 180
Cholesterol, 52–53
Chronic illness, 16
Cognitive restructuring, 133–134
Conditionally essential amino acids, 6
Contingency management, 134–136
c-reactive protein, 54

Decisional balance questions, 128, 129
Diet
  low-carbohydrate diets
    antioxidants and phytochemicals, 102
    benefits, 101–102
    carbohydrate intake, 100
    glycogen depletion, 100
    ketosis, 100
    patient populations, 105
    physical activity and exercise, 101
    plant-based diet, 103–104
  Mexican diet, 32
  moderate and low-fat diets
    acceptable macronutrient distribution range, 95
    animal fats, 96
    benefits, 97–98

caloric deficit, 99
DASH diet, 95
low-calorie fruits and vegetables, 95
nutritional adequacy, 99
one-day menu, 96–97
plant-based fats, 95
saturated fat, 95
VLCD (*See* Very low calorie diet (VLCD))
Dietary Approaches to Stop Hypertension (DASH), 95
Dietary behavior modification
cognitive restructuring, 133–134
contingency management, 134–136
environmental considerations
location, 140–141
people, 139–140
goal setting, 131–132
motivational interviewing
affirmation statement, 130
alcoholics, 128
decisional balance questions, 128, 129
goal, 128
open-ended questions, 128, 129
patient's self-efficay, 129
reflection statements, 129–130
problem-solving, 132–133
self-monitoring, 127–128
stress management, 137–139
structured meal plans, 130–131
Dietary intake
food frequency questionnaires, 59–60
food records, 58–59
twenty-four hour dietary recalls, 57–58
Diethylpropion, 151
Disaccharide polymers, 3

Energy balance, 6
Essential amino acids, 6

Fats, 4–5
FFQ. *See* Food frequency questionnaires
Food frequency questionnaires (FFQ), 59–60

Growth charts, 43

Infantometer, 43

Ketosis, 100

LAGB. *See* Laparoscopic adjustable gastric banding
Laparoscopic adjustable gastric banding (LAGB), 165–167
Laproscopic sleeve gastrectomy, 163–164
Leptin deficiency, 25
Linolenic acid, 5
Liraglutide, 149–150
Long-term diet, 172–173
Lorcaserin, 146–147

Macronutrient, 105–106
Medications
benzphetamine, 150–151
diethylpropion, 151
liraglutide, 149–150
lorcaserin, 146–147
naltrexone and bupropion, 153
orlistat, 147–149
phentermine, 145–146, 151–153
topiramate, 151–153
Mental health, 17
MI. *See* Motivational interviewing
Monosaccharide polymers, 3
Monounsaturated fats, 4
Motivational interviewing (MI)
affirmation statement, 130
alcoholics, 128
decisional balance questions, 128, 129
goal, 128
open-ended questions, 128, 129
patient's self-efficay, 129
reflection statements, 129–130

Naltrexone, 153
National Health and Nutrition Examination Survey (NHANES), 11
NHANES. *See* National Health and Nutrition Examination Survey

Nonessential amino acids, 6
Nutritional counseling, 160–162
Nutrition assessment
  biochemical indicators
    cholesterol, 52–53
    c-reactive protein, 54
    glucose and associated indicators, 51–52
    reference values, 54
    uric acid, 53
  body fat, 49–50
  body mass index
    bed scales, 45
    children's growth charts, 43
    classifications, 45–46
    Frankfort horizontal plane, 42
    infantometer, 43
    limitation, 41
    patient's height and weight, 42
    pediatric pan scale, 44
    stadiometer, 42
    standing position, 44
    standing scale, 44
    vertical height, 43
    weight status, 42
    wheelchair scales, 45
    WHO Growth Charts, 46
  dietary intake
    food frequency questionnaires, 59–60
    food records, 58–59
    twenty-four hour dietary recalls, 57–58
  food beliefs and preferences, 62–63
  historical data, 60–62
  physical signs and symptoms
    acanthosis nigricans, 56
    blood pressure, 55
    body shape, 55–56
    physical finding, 56
  waist circumference
    cosmetic pencil, 47
    gender, 48
    nonstretch measuring tape, 47
    waist-to-stature ratios, 48
Nutrition education
  empty calorie foods
    caloric deficit, 112
    foods and beverages, 111
    instructional ideas, 112–113
  meal frequency, 120–121
  meal replacements, 121–123
  nutrition facts labels, 115–116
  planning and preparing meals
    food preparation and cooking equipment, 118
    food preparation methods, 119–120
    recommendation, 117
  portion control, concept of, 113–115

Obesity
  cancer, 15–16
  cardiovascular disease, 13–14
  chronic illness, 16
  disparities, 12–13
  interpersonal factors
    cultural factors, 32–33
    food and physical activity environments, 33–34
    social networks, 31–32
    workplaces and schools, 34–35
  mental health, 17
  modifiable risk factors
    attitudes and beliefs, 27–28
    diet and physical activity-related behaviors, 28–30
    knowledge, 26–27
    psychological disturbances, 30–31
  non-modifiable risk factors
    family history, 24
    genetics, 24–26
  prevalence, 11–12
  type 2 diabetes mellitus, 14–15
Oligosaccharides, 4
Omega 3 fatty acid, 5
Open-ended questions, 128, 129
Orlistat, 147–149

Patient's self-efficacy, 129
Pediatric pan scale, 44
Phentermine, 145–146, 151–153
Physical activity
  federal guidelines, 177–178

food intake, 181
mental health, 180–181
physical activity plan, 178
physical health outcomes, 179–180
weight status and body composition, 178–179
Phytochemicals, 102
Plant-based diet, 103–104
Plant-based fats, 95
Polysaccharide polymers, 4
Prader-Willi syndrome, 25

RDN. *See* Registered Dietitian Nutritionist
REE. *See* Resting energy expenditure
Registered Dietitian Nutritionist (RDN), 57, 70, 73, 84, 160
Resting energy expenditure (REE), 81
Roux-en-Y Gastric Bypass, 164–165

Saturated fat, 95
Self-monitoring, 127–128
Set point theory, 8
SMART. *See* Specific, measurable, achievable, realistic, and timely
Social networks, 31–32
Specific, measurable, achievable, realistic, and timely (SMART) goals, 86, 88
Stress management, 137–139
Structured meal plans, 130–131

Topiramate, 151–153
Trans fats, 4
Type 2 diabetes mellitus, 14–15

Unsaturated fats, 4
Uric acid, 53
U.S. Food and Drug Administration, 2

Very low calorie diet (VLCD)
benefits, 92
bowel habits, 93
complications and side effects, 94
coping strategies, 93
fatigue and tiredness, 93
meal replacements, 91
nausea and diarrhea, 94
regular dietary guidance and support, 93
VLCD. *See* Very low calorie diet

Weight loss surgery
biliopancreatic diversion with duodenal switch (BDB/DS), 167
laparoscopic adjustable gastric banding, 165–167
laproscopic sleeve gastrectomy, 163–164
postoperative nutrition therapy
bariatric soft diet, 171–172
clear and full liquids, 167–169
long-term diet, 172–173
supplementation, 169–170
preoperative care
medical clearance, 158–160
nutritional counseling, 160–162
psychological evaluation, 162
Roux-en-Y Gastric Bypass, 164–165
surgical criteria, 157–158
Weight management programs
behavioral modification, 73
behavior modification, 80
biochemical factors, 80
caloric goals
adults, 82–84
children, 84
calorie, 79
dietary component, 72–73
early intervention, 74
frequency and duration, 75
health status, 80
mental health goals, 80
multidisciplinary team, 70–71
patient, 69–70
patient energy
children, 82
indirect calorimetry, 81
physical activity factor, 81
resting energy expenditure (REE), 81
TEE calculations, 82
patient's blood pressure, 80

patient's dietary intake and physical activity habits, 80
physical activity component, 73
physical and mental health, 80
Registered Dietitian Nutritionist, 70
scheduling considerations, 75–76
SMART, behavioral goals, 86, 88
supporters, 72
target weight
  adults, 84–85
  children, 85–86
WHO Growth Charts, 46

OTHER TITLES IN OUR NUTRITION AND DIETETICS PRACTICE COLLECTION

Katie Ferraro, University of San Francisco School of Nursing, Editor

Nutrition Support
by Brenda O'Day

Diet and Disease: Nutrition for Heart Disease, Diabetes, and Metabolic Stress
by Katie Ferraro

Diet and Disease: Nutrition for Gastrointestinal, Musculoskeletal, Hepatobiliary, Pancreatic, and Kidney Diseases
by Katie Ferraro

FORTHCOMING TITLES FOR THIS COLLECTION

Introduction to Dietetic Practice
by Katie Ferraro

Dietary Supplements
by B. Bryan Haycock and Amy A. Sunderman

Sports Nutrition
by Kary Woodruff

www.ingramcontent.com/pod-product-compliance
Lightning Source LLC
LaVergne TN
LVHW052324200926
848481LV00002B/659
9781606507636